The Complete Idiot's Reference Card

Thirteen Things You Can Do to Grow Younger Starting *Now*

1. Engage in vigorous physi... ...as taking the stairs instead of the eleva...

2. Start cutting down on al... ...diet. Don't worry: You'll have *plenty* ... ...th-filled Youth Foods™ you will be eati...

3. Drink freshly squeezed fruit and veget... ...s is in addition to abundant water.

4. Keep abreast of new developments in age-reversal and longevity. Experiment and enjoy.

5. Sunscreen isn't enough to keep your skin looking young. Wear hats and light covering in strong sunlight.

6. Dry brush your skin every single day. That keeps it glowing.

7. Treat yourself to regular massages. Massage is a luxury that's a necessity.

8. Bring your look up to date. Treat yourself to a new hairstyle and wardrobe.

9. Study something new ... a new language, swing dancing, a musical instrument, singing in a chorus.

10. Don't expect your attitudes toward aging to change overnight. Remember, Rome wasn't destroyed in a day.

11. Keep your spirits up in the face of setbacks. Use obstacles for motivation.

12. Always remember: You're never too old to make really dramatic changes.

13. Whatever you do, make it an adventure.

Sallie's and Hattie's Four-Step E.A.S.E. Road to Youth

E = EXERCISE to feel fabulous forever

Fitness is the first step.

A = ATTITUDES that keep you young

Change your thinking; change your aging.

S = SKINCARE means treating it right

Head-to-toe care keeps you smooth and sexy.

E = EATING—it's not just a matter of weight

What's on your plate can seal your fate.

alpha books

Twenty-Five Hattietudes™ for a Young Attitude

- ➤ Never forget the YOU in YOUTH!
- ➤ Your first youth is a gift from Mother Nature; your second is a gift from yourself.
- ➤ Faith is the mortar of optimism.
- ➤ Optimism is the foundation of youth.
- ➤ Aging changes the "ME" Generation into RE-generation.
- ➤ Age is never the reason … it's the excuse.
- ➤ Remember: IMPOSSIBLE = I'M POSSIBLE.
- ➤ The opposite of Old isn't Young, it's NEW.
- ➤ The path to youth is paved with possibility.
- ➤ Convert envy into inspiration, and you'll never run out of fuel.
- ➤ Age doesn't make you forget—it teaches you what's important to remember.
- ➤ Fighting Mother Nature is good exercise.
- ➤ Wrinkles don't make you old. Infants have plenty of them.
- ➤ Never give up your dreams. They keep you awake.
- ➤ Beauty is never just skin deep.
- ➤ Don't let gravity get you down.
- ➤ Keep climbing, and you'll never be over the hill.
- ➤ When life gets harder, you get smarter.
- ➤ The hands of time belong to you. Take aging into your own hands.
- ➤ Love is contagious. Go out and start an epidemic.
- ➤ Self-hatred doesn't come naturally; it's an acquired taste.
- ➤ Both blame and shame maim.
- ➤ Suffering is an option you don't have to pick up.
- ➤ If you were sexy when you were young, you'll be even sexier when you're older.
- ➤ Youth isn't wasted on the young—or on anyone else!

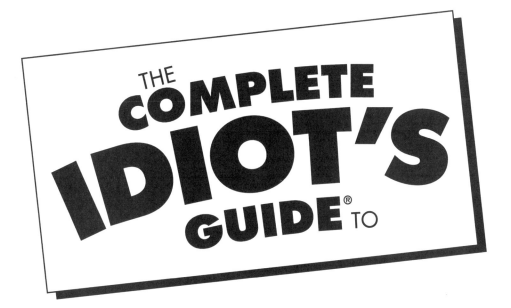

THE **COMPLETE IDIOT'S GUIDE®** TO

Looking and Feeling Younger

by Sallie Batson and Hattie

alpha books

Macmillan USA, Inc.
201 West 103rd Street
Indianapolis, IN 46290

A Pearson Education Company

International Standard Book Number: 0-02-863923-5
Library of Congress Catalog Card Number: Available upon request.

02 01 00   8 7 6 5 4 3 2 1

Interpretation of the printing code: The rightmost number of the first series of numbers is the year of the book's printing; the rightmost number of the second series of numbers is the number of the book's printing. For example, a printing code of 00-1 shows that the first printing occurred in 2000.

Printed in the United States of America

Publisher
Marie Butler-Knight

Product Manager
Phil Kitchel

Managing Editor
Cari Luna

Senior Acquisitions Editor
Renee Wilmeth

Development Editor
Amy Gordon

Production Editor
Christy Wagner

Copy Editor
Fran Blauw

Illustrator
Jody Schaeffer

Cover Designers
Mike Freeland
Kevin Spear

Book Designers
Scott Cook and Amy Adams of DesignLab

Indexer
Amy Lawrence

Layout/Proofreading
Angela Calvert
John Etchison
Wendy Ott

Contents at a Glance

Appendixes

Contents

Foreword

You're about to embark on an exciting and informative adventure. If you've ever worried about growing older, as most of us have, it's amazing how the first image that comes to mind when we think of aging involves loss of vitality as time robs us of the ability to do all the fun things we love.

How long our parents and grandparents lived is only *slightly* indicative of our life expectancy. In fact, genes account for very little when projecting how long and how well we will live. Aging is definitely in the eye—and the attitude—of the beholder.

Americans are living longer than ever. A hundred years ago—at the start of the twentieth century—the average lifespan was only 47. Now it's 77, and 47 is the age when most of us are finally reaching success in so many areas of life.

This longevity raises new questions that need to be addressed and answered: Does living longer mean that we'll automatically become old and infirm? What can we do to keep our bodies from losing flexibility and energy? Are loss of memory, muscle tone, physical stamina, and sex drive inevitable? Most important, what can be done for us to look and feel younger at 50, 60, 70, ... even 80, 90, or 100?

Every one of us knows people who see their thirtieth birthday as the start of middle age and those who are old at 40. We also know others who are young and alive well into their 80s and 90s. These people have grown in wisdom, all the while remaining active in body, mind, and spirit.

Marcel Proust wrote "The true voyage of self-discovery lies not in seeking new landscapes but in having new eyes." Use these new eyes to see what's ahead and what's possible when we begin to grow younger as we age.

Sallie and Hattie came together to write about reversing aging from different backgrounds. Sallie is a journalist researching and reporting health and lifestyle matters—including how we age—while writing for newspapers and magazines as well as books. Hattie, who at various times has been a dance teacher, psychotherapist, and bodywork expert, began her journey as a personal quest to remain young and fit. This is their second book together, validating and furthering their commitment to altering how we all view the way we age and what *anyone* can do to remain youthful for as long as possible.

Together, they share a wealth of practical measures that *anyone* can incorporate into their lives that will help retard, even reverse, aging.

I enthusiastically look forward to this adventure.

Julie Wilson

Julie Wilson is the quintessential cabaret singer. She has been a glittering star in the nightclub scene for many years. Stephen Holden wrote in *The New York Times*, "Julie Wilson has established herself as the most elegant and fiercely expressive singer-actress on New York's cabaret circuit ... unmatched by her peers." She starred in Broadway's *Kismet, The Pajama Game, Jimmy,* and *Legs Diamond,* which won her a Tony nomination. She toured in *Kiss Me, Kate* and originated the role of Bianca in the London production. Miss Wilson has won numerous awards from the Mable Mercer Foundation at Town Hall, the Manhattan Association of Cabarets and Clubs, and the USO.

Introduction

Remember when you were 12 and couldn't wait until you were old enough to drive a car ... or go to girl-and-boy parties? You'd have your own money, and no one could tell you when to go to bed. And when you were in high school, remember how impatient you were to go to college or get a job? You were sure everything would be great once you were a Grown-Up.

Of course everything changed once you hit 25 ... or 30 ... or even 50 ... and you realized that you were no longer that child fantasizing about the future. Suddenly, you were the Grown-Up, and you felt old.

Nobody wants to be old (shudder). Just turn on the TV or check the magazine covers, and you'll see the catch phrases: Anti-Aging. Age-Reversal. Age-Defying. So what's a person to do?

You'll find the answers here, in *The Complete Idiot's Guide to Looking and Feeling Younger*.

This book is designed to help you transform both your mind and your body so that you become more youthful with each passing year. It zeros in on any negative internal conversation you may have about aging and turns it around to accommodate a new way of aging fit for the twenty-first century. This combined physical, mental, and spiritual approach holds the key to a life of vitality, sexuality, and ongoing renewal.

Step by step, you will learn ...

> ➤ Not only how to slow down the aging process, but also how to actually reverse it.

> ➤ To be more fit, healthy, and vital than ever before, regardless of your age.

> ➤ To transform your thinking about aging so that you experience it as an adventure, an opportunity, and a gift.

> ➤ To look and feel at least 10 years younger.

The Complete Idiot's Guide to Looking and Feeling Younger gives you a unique and highly effective program to turn your devitalizing beliefs and unhealthy habits into life-altering ones. Transforming your thinking not only leads to better self-care practices but also helps modify the aging process itself. What you once might have considered negative experiences you will now see as chances for growth. This reduces your stress level, enhances your sense of well-being, and radically delays the aging process.

It is a statistical reality that for the first time in history, people have a good possibility of living full and productive lives well into their 90s. With advances in technology, superb body care, and this positive way of viewing aging, you can give yourself the miracle of a long, healthy life. And, may we add, an exciting and sexual one at that.

For most of us, old age is perceived as both negative and inevitable. We may hate it or make our peace with it, but nevertheless, it is viewed as a necessary evil. Sure, it may bring wisdom and maturity (how often do you hear "Youth is wasted on the young" or "If I knew then what I know now"?), but compared to the appealing qualities of youth, old age seems to fall seriously short.

How often have we dreamed about how great it would be if we could have both the attributes of youth and age?

We believe this to be entirely possible. In fact, our lives are dedicated to this quest. We have discovered the secrets to growing young with the passage of years rather than passively accepting the ravages of time.

In this book, we happily share them with you. What we have come to understand is that no matter how old you are, if you decide to commit yourself to being vital in mind, body, and spirit, you will achieve lifelong youthfulness.

When we are young, nature takes care of us. We have boundless energy, unending curiosity, the ability to learn rapidly, and infinite flexibility—and we are usually quite adorable. With age, nature seems to say, "You're on your own now, kid."

And we are.

Rather than feel distraught and abandoned, we can use this fact as a source of inspiration and self-respect. We realize that we can finally fashion our lives according to our desires and dreams. We can shape our present and our future. That is the lesson aging teaches us. Our lives belong to us in the sense that we have control over how and who we are—the outcome is based on the decisions we make.

We need not fear the loss of youth simply because time is passing. With courage, hard work, faith, and love, each of us can live a life that is truly fulfilling.

Is it a difficult challenge? Yes, it certainly is.

Is it a miraculous adventure? Without doubt.

We invite you to be part of a new generation that embraces aging as a glorious opportunity to live a life resplendent with dignity and delight.

How to Use This Book

We've divided *The Complete Idiot's Guide to Looking and Feeling Younger* into six parts. First, we guide you through a personal assessment of your body and how you feel about the way you are aging. Then we provide you with exciting and effective techniques to keep you young for your entire life.

You can enjoy reading this book from cover to cover, like we wrote it, or check out the table of contents and jump to any topic that appeals to you. Whatever you decide, make it fun.

Part 1, "Here's Looking at You," starts you off with a full assessment of your body—your overall health; your skin, mouth, and hair; how and what you eat; and how much exercise you're getting. Looking at yourself this closely prepares you for your age-reversing adventure.

Part 2, "Taking a Look at Youth," leads you through three aspects of staying young. The first explores how thoughts—both negative and positive—influence the aging process. The second teaches you to create an environment that surrounds you with youth, and the third introduces simple ways to update your appearance.

Part 3, "Looking and Feeling Young with E.A.S.E.," is the heart of our age-reversing program. E stands for Exercise, A for Attitude, S for Skincare, and the final E for Eating. Mastering these four steps will give you the tools to create a life of vitality and glowing health.

Part 4, "Putting Youth on Your Plate," expands on the "E for Eating" part of your E.A.S.E. program. You'll learn how to combine food and eat a diet high in Super Dense Nutrients (SDNs). Changing a lifetime of destructive eating habits will help you look and feel younger, thinner, and healthier. You'll also get a full discussion of supplements to help reverse aging.

Part 5, "Dear Doctor," delves into the rich array of alternatives to traditional medicine, such as acupuncture and homeopathy. You'll also learn about Mother Nature's apothecary and what foods, herbs, spices, and essential oils can enhance your plan to transform your life. Finally, you'll look at the advantages cosmetic surgery and dental innovations can offer.

Part 6, "Living a Life You Love," gives you the inspiration to create a future that enriches you personally and contributes to humanity. It delves into your deepest dreams and provides you with an extraordinary opportunity to fulfill them.

Young Ideas

Sprinkled throughout the book are tidbits of information written to jump off the page. These sidebars highlight special information that makes your quest to look and feel younger interesting and fun.

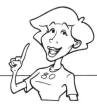

Voice of Experience

We've dipped into history, our teachers, therapists, and friends to bring you nuggets of wisdom that refresh the spirit and enrich the mind.

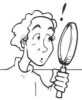

Age Alert

These are things you should know before you head off-course. After all, we don't want you to get older before you finish the book!

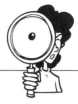

WatchWord

You'll find definitions of new words and concepts in these boxes. They'll help you to expand your understanding of aging and what to do about reversing it.

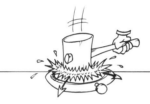

Time Stopper

There is so much you can do to slow the aging process. We've highlighted many of these tips to speed you along your path.

Acknowledgements

We extend our heartfelt thanks to our expert resources—Dr. Gerry Herman, Dr. Dana G. Cohen, Patsy Roth, Colin Lively, Dr. Richard Marfuggi, Joel Benjamin, Dr. John Kildahl, Dr. Viana Muller, Dr. Alan Cohen, Lou Bartfield, Patricia Betty, Shawne Mitchell, Helen Lee, Ila Brody, Laura Geller, Louis Price, Jim Graham, Pamela Rice, Priscilla Averbuck, Joshua Wiener, Eve Robinson, Sandye Pinz, Joy Pierson, Bart Potenza, Gautam Mukerji, Dr. John Juhl, Richard Downs, Bill Miller, Madeline Kaplan, Larry Jacobs, Hilda and Michael Meltzer, Mr. Joe Franklin, and his medical sidekick, Dr. Jonathan D. Silver—for their contributions to our work. You have inspired us beyond measure.

We both extend our thanks and appreciation to all who shared their wisdom with us so that we could share it with you. Particular thanks to our most caring agent, Sheree Bykofsky, and her energetic associate, Janet Rosen, and to our ever-supportive, eagle-eyed editors, Renee Wilmeth, Amy Gordon, Christy Wagner, and Fran Blauw. It takes countless individuals to make a book such as this come together. We thank you all.

From Hattie: I acknowledge Werner Erhard for helping me create the possibility of RetroAge® and for the privilege of working with my beloved writing partner, Sallie Batson. I am blessed by all whose lives have touched mine for the trust, beauty, and love you've provided.

Trademarks

Part 1

Here's Looking at You

Most of us have a pretty good idea of what we weigh … and what we wish we weighed. We also know how tall we are. After all, we had to tell the guy at the DMV our height and weight to get a driver's license. We know the size of the last item of clothing we bought and whether it pinches at the waist. And we can describe the cut or color of our hair and countless other aspects of our appearance.

What we don't know is the true condition of our bodies—inside and out—especially with regard to aging. We were going along quite nicely and, suddenly, one morning, we couldn't recognize that old person staring back at us in the mirror.

Part 1 introduces you to that person and, in doing so, guides you in charting your journey to lifelong youth. But before that happens, you need to know where you are when you begin. So let's take inventory of your current condition.

Throughout this part, you will consider the question "Are you as young as you want to be?" We often avoid making such assessments and may be reluctant to answer questions and make lists. We've posed these questions to help you define every aspect of aging right at the onset.

Then you'll be ready to look and feel younger—starting now.

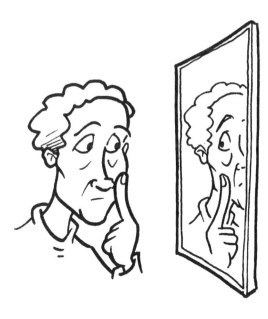

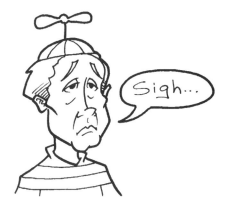

Chapter 1

Are You as Young as You Want to Be?

In This Chapter

➤ Getting started getting younger

➤ Nipping aging in the bud

➤ Taking an honest look at your body

➤ Giving yourself the once-over

➤ Why a *BodyCheck?*

Picasso had the right idea when he said "It takes a long time to become young."

To that we add "You're never too old to become young." All you need is the desire and the dedication to create a body that radiates youth and then to design a life that matches it. By the time you've finished this book, you'll have what it takes to look and feel at least 10 years younger.

Many 50-plussers have expressed the sentiment that they feel more energetic and to-gether now than they did in their 30s. It's a matter of perspective, they say. What seemed so significant and threatening at 30 is incidental at 50.

Still, although attitudes and interests can remain youthful, bodies often show wear and tear with time. The trick is to face the physical condition of your body as it is right now and then use this information to transform how you age. Even simple steps will make an immediate difference in halting this process so that you start looking and feeling younger in no time at all.

Catch Those Early Signs

It's far from impossible. The process starts as soon as you make the decision to take aging into your own hands. When you realize that nature and time have taken over and you don't like what you see in the mirror, you're ready to begin.

Catch those early signs of aging—spider veins, wrinkles, dry patches, even hair sprouting where you wish it wouldn't—and nip them in the bud. You won't be able to do that if you're not aware of what's going on. That's why we ask you to start paying attention to even the smallest details.

The first step toward making any change is to know where to begin. That's why we've created a complete inventory of the State of Your Body—a *BodyCheck*—for you to fill out.

Time Stopper

When you realize that the face you see in the mirror isn't the face you see in your mind, you're ready to stop aging and start growing younger.

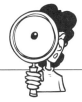

WatchWord

Every time you see the word **BodyCheck,** you'll be asked to observe the condition of your body and how you feel about it at that precise moment so that you can monitor each step of your age-reversing process.

Taking an Honest Look at Your Body

Now is the time to record your vital statistics. Don't be afraid to be honest. You don't have to shave off those 10 pounds you picked up over the holidays … or say your waist is four inches smaller than it actually is. You'll be the only one to see these numbers.

Several basic questionnaires follow that are designed to not only unearth information about your current physical condition but to put you in touch with how you feel about your body. Notice that, although most of the blanks ask for simple statistics, we've thrown in some highly subjective questions. These are not traps to trip you up. Rather, they are keys to open the truth about how you experience your body and how aging has affected it.

The best way to approach this process is to answer the BodyCheck questions as truthfully and objectively as you can.

When assessing your posture and flexibility, we recommend that you stand in front of a full-length mirror. You'll also want a stable chair or table to use for balance.

How Well Are You?

Most of us rarely think about the various systems or parts of our bodies. We either feel well or we don't. This BodyCheck will put an end to all that generalizing. It is designed to determine exactly how you perceive your body's present physical condition. It will not diagnose disease, although it may make you aware of problems you may have ignored.

Fill in the specifics where called for. Where a subjective response is needed, just write what immediately comes to mind. For example, your assessment of your muscle tone might be "Calves great, thighs not. Arms weak." Other items, such as Fluid Retention, Menopause, Impotency, Ability to Heal, and Cold Hands and Feet, might make you aware of some conditions you have avoided facing. Here's your chance to do something about them and perhaps even discuss them with your health care professional.

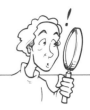

Age Alert

Don't skip over the written exercises. They're not homework to be graded. You'll find a lot of knowledge in your answers, so fill them in now and enjoy the process of getting to know yourself.

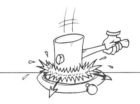

Time Stopper

Sometimes filling out forms is no fun at all. And looking in the mirror from all angles can be daunting. Now's the time to move past this resistance and just do it! It'll be worth it.

BodyCheck

Take inventory of your entire body and the way it functions so you can have an idea of your level of overall well-being.

Name: _____ Date: 9-22-00

Actual age: 54 _____ Age you look: 50 _____

Smoker: NO ___ Drinker: NO ___ Drug User: NO ___

Height: 5' 5" _____ More/less than at age 20: _____

Posture (standing, walking, sitting): _____

Actual weight: 190 _____ Desired weight: 140 _____

Able/unable to maintain desired weight: _____

Pounds you want to gain or lose: 50 _____

Measurements:

Bust: _____ Waist: _____ Hips: _____

Unwanted fat (how much and where): _____

Overall muscle tone (rate on scale of 1 to 10, 10 being ideal): _____

Energy level (rate on scale of 1 to 10, 10 being ideal): _____

Flexibility

(Range of motion in all joints)

Rate 1 to 10, with 10 being full mobility without pain.

Fingers: _____ Wrists: _____ Elbows: _____

Arm: Forward: _____ Backward: _____ Up: _____

Shoulder rotation:

   Right— Forward: _____ Backward: _____

   Left— Forward: _____ Backward: _____

Neck:

   Side to side: _____ Forward/backward: _____ Circular rotation: _____

Back:

Upper back/waist:

   Side to side: _____ Forward/backward: _____ Circular rotation: _____

Lower back/pelvis:

   Side to side: _____ Forward/backward: _____ Circular rotation: _____

Legs *(hold on to something stable for balance while doing these):*

—Extend leg and lift.

   Right— Forward: _____ Side to side: _____

   Left— Forward: _____ Side to side: _____

Knee:

—Bend leg backward to flex knee.

   Right— Forward: _____ Side to side: _____

   Left— Forward: _____ Side to side: _____

Ankles *(sit while checking these joints):*

   Right— Flex: _____ Point: _____ Rotate: _____

   Left— Flex: _____ Point: _____ Rotate: _____

Chronic pains:

   Where: _____ For how long: _____

   Where: _____ For how long: _____

   Where: _____ For how long: _____

6

Immune System

(Note frequency of recurrence)

Infections: _____

Ability of wounds to heal: _____

Allergies: _____

Hayfever: _____

Sinus congestion: _____

Cold/flu: _____

Bronchitis: _____

Congestion: _____

Sore throat/tonsillitis: _____

Laryngitis: _____

Migraine headaches: _____

Stress level: _____

Sugar cravings: _____

Blood-sugar irregularities: _____

Circulatory System

High/low blood pressure: _____

Heart disease: _____

Cholesterol level: _____

Triglyceride level: _____

Cold hands/feet: _____

Numbness/tingling: _____

Varicose veins: _____

Spider veins: _____

Lightheadedness: _____

Dizziness: _____

Digestive System/Elimination

(Frequency or extent of condition)

Ulcers: _____

Indigestion: _____

Heartburn: _____

"Nervous stomach": _____

Diarrhea: _____

Constipation: _____

Bloating: _____

Fluid retention: _____

Frequent urination: _____

Painful urination: _____

Slow/fast metabolism: _____

Anorexia: _____

Bulimia: _____

Reproductive System

Women

Menstruation/regularity: _____   Age at onset: _____

Premenstrual Syndrome (PMS): _____

Pregnancies: _____

Number of children: _____

Infertility: _____

Menopause (age began): _____

Men

Impotence (age began/frequency): _____

Prostate dysfunction: _____

Nervous System/Emotions

Hyperactivity: _____

Hypoactivity: _____

Adverse reactions to stress: _____

Anxiety: _____

Depression: _____

Bipolar disorder: _____

Mood swings: _____

Fatigue: _____

Stamina: _____

Vision

Nearsighted/farsighted/astigmatic: _____

Colorblindness: _____

Glasses/contact lenses: _____ Bi/trifocals: _____ How long: _____

Glaucoma: _____ Cataracts: _____

Conjunctivitis: _____ Frequency: _____

Other conditions: _____

Hearing

Hearing loss: _____

Degree of loss: _____

Correction: _____

Tinnitus (ringing in the ears): _____

Pain: _____ Discharge: _____ Wax: _____

Infections (frequency): _____

Do you work in an environment with a high noise level (music studio, factory, construction site, etc.)? _____

Overview

Chronic illnesses:

What: _____ For how long: _____

What: _____ For how long: _____

What: _____ For how long: _____

What: _____ For how long: _____

Hospitalizations/surgeries:

What: _____ For how long: _____

What: _____ For how long: _____

What: _____ For how long: _____

What: _____ For how long: _____

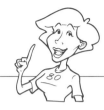

Voice of Experience

"How old would you be if you didn't know how old you were?"

—Anonymous

How Did It Feel to Take This Inventory?

As we were writing this, we wondered if it would be challenging in a positive or a negative way for you to fill out this inventory. Naturally, it was our intention to have you face yourself fully and honestly to begin the necessary steps to start growing younger.

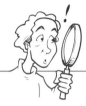

Age Alert

If you have trouble visualizing what 10 or 15 pounds looks like so you can identify how many pounds you need to lose or how much you have already lost, ask a butcher to show you a piece of meat of the equivalent weight. Or, if you're a vegetarian, weigh out 10 pounds of fruit. If that's not possible, or you can't wait for the market to open, a standard telephone weighs about four pounds; a healthy four-year-old child weighs about 40.

When we started our own age-reversal programs, we were hesitant to look at all facets of our aging. Some we chose to ignore … until it was no longer possible, while others we attacked with zest.

Take desired weight, for example: By admitting how much we wish we really weighed, we would be forced to change how we ate. Not a welcome prospect, to say the least.

Sallie has battled pounds for most of her adult life. She had begun to accept her body in its overweight state until she reconnected with her desire to be fit and healthy. Facing the condition of her body rekindled her hope for a more youthful, trim figure. An effective diet and exercise plan followed, along with a substantial weight loss.

Hattie wasn't the least bit hesitant to study herself in the mirror. As a dance/exercise teacher and now an age-reversing expert, she is completely at ease with her naked body—even with its flaws. What bothered her was having to admit that her beloved hours on the beaches of the Caribbean seriously damaged her skin. On the negative side, she was forced to curtail this pleasure. On the positive side, she created some extraordinary techniques for reversing sun damage that she shares later in this book.

Now what about you? Did this BodyCheck empower you, or were you discouraged? If you were discouraged, we suggest that you turn that around and learn to use your negativity to inspire you.

If you find that your arms are weak and flabby, just think how much more you'll be able to do after you tone up this problem area—like being able to pick up your grandchildren with ease, engaging in new hobbies, and participating in exciting new activities that you always wanted to try but couldn't. And if you're very overweight, even though you may find it depressing to see it in the mirror, you can use this image as a "before shot" to see how far you've come once the weight starts coming off.

We also suggest that if you had trouble filling out the form and answering the questions, just put it aside for now and come back to it later. Or better yet, just fill in the spaces you feel comfortable with and leave the rest blank for another time.

Just the act of reading through the questions can make a difference in awakening your awareness of your body.

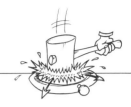

Time Stopper

If weight loss is your goal, every morning before you start your day, and every evening at bedtime, stand in front of your full-length mirror and say your target weight out loud. Repeat it 10 times ... with conviction.

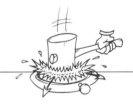

Time Stopper

Facing yourself keeps getting easier as you see positive changes happening. Don't give up!

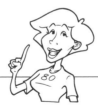

Voice of Experience

It can be uncomfortable, even scary, to deal with illness and aging. The fastest way to diffuse these fears is to acknowledge them. It's amazing how quickly they dissipate when you stare them in the face.

Was This BodyCheck Necessary? You Bet!

So why did we ask for a complete BodyCheck now? Usually we only take inventory of our bodies when we suspect that something is wrong, if we're changing doctors, or we're joining a new gym (they want to know about your physical condition to protect themselves and their liability insurance). In this case, you did it to get a true picture of your state of health.

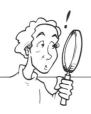

Age Alert

Most people tend to treat themselves with less care as they get older. Just because we're no longer babies in need of a parent's care doesn't mean we don't deserve TLC. We certainly do, so make sure you get lots of it.

It's impossible to be youthful without being healthy. We cannot stress this point enough. Youth and vitality are inseparable from good health. You can't have one without the other. You may look dynamite, dress fantastically, and have every material benefit on the planet—but unless your body is fit and in good health, no amount of money or makeup can make you look truly young.

Now we don't want to discourage you from doing your best to look and dress wonderfully. These things are certainly important. We simply want to drive home the necessity of diligent focus on the care of the body to keep you on target for life.

The Least You Need to Know

➤ To create a youth-filled future, you must be aware of where you are right now.

➤ Your feelings about age and aging help determine how young or old you look.

➤ Be absolutely truthful about your present physical condition. You aren't being graded.

➤ Facing imperfections is the first step toward correcting them.

➤ Health and youth go hand in hand.

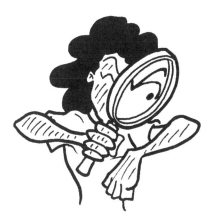

How Old Does Your Skin Look?

In This Chapter

➤ Detecting early signs of aging

➤ Defining common flaws

➤ Charting your skin

➤ Assessing how you feel about your skin

➤ Measuring your makeup style—young or old?

Like it or not, the first signs of aging often show up on the skin.

One morning as you're mindlessly brushing your teeth, the sight of a web of tiny wrinkles suddenly rivets your attention to the area around your eyes. Surely they weren't there yesterday. Ah, old age has arrived; now these tiny lines are all you can see.

Yes, lines and wrinkles can erode our faces and bodies as we grow older, but there's a lot that can be done to halt, and even reverse, their seeming inevitability.

Exquisite, young-looking skin is one of our most prized possessions. When our skin is wonderful, we feel wonderful. Conversely, when our skin looks blotchy or feels dry and scaly, we are haunted by how old we appear. And we are frightened that it will keep getting worse.

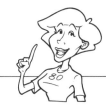

Voice of Experience

According to makeup consultant Laura Geller, who beautifies women of all ages in New York's Laura Geller Makeup Studios, "For every night you don't take off your mascara, you age two weeks."

Your Skin Says It All

Everything that is wrong with your health will show up on your skin. It is the body's largest organ. You must educate yourself to be super alert to its texture, tone, and quality. This awareness will help you create and maintain a state of radiant health.

And with radiant health comes lasting youth.

Never let a day go by without rubbing, kneading, or briskly massaging your body, including your feet, hands, and scalp. The more stimulation you provide your skin, the more healthy and glowing it becomes. While animals have fur and fish have scales, we humans have only a light covering of hair and our clothing to protect us. Unless we give our skin the attention it needs, it will grow ugly and old-looking. Nobody wants that.

Your skin is the boundary between yourself and the world. If it is healthy and well cared for, it will protect and provide for you for a lifetime. Everybody wants that.

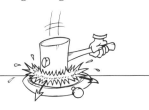

Time Stopper

The more you touch your skin, the more touchable it becomes.

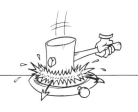

Time Stopper

There is no way to be youthful without making sure that you take superb care of your skin. A day of neglecting your skin is a day you're adding to your age.

Signs of the Times

It doesn't matter what shape your skin is in when you begin this assessment. As we delve into age-reversing techniques later in this book, you will learn how to regenerate your skin so that it looks and feels younger and more alive each day, regardless of how it looks at this moment.

Before you can reclaim the soft and supple skin of your youth, you need to be aware of its present condition. Once again, we ask you to complete a full BodyCheck. This time it will be of your skin so that you have a clear picture of how it is aging.

Get out that full-length mirror and bright light, strip down, and get ready to check yourself out—front and back, head to toe. You'll need a hand mirror—or even a friend—to study your back and to locate those hidden places you'd rather not have to look at in the first place.

What You're Looking For

Skin damage takes a variety of forms, be it a scar from a childhood fall in the park, stretch marks from pregnancy, or knee surgery from a football injury. Regrettably, the most insidious youth stealer to plague our skin is the sun. Damage done to the skin in childhood can cause serious problems—such as skin cancer—in adulthood if we don't take steps to correct it.

If you're like most folks, you hardly pay attention to your skin unless you have a sunburn, rash, or cut. If you're planning to grow younger, and we're sure you are, you'll have to learn to be aware of every possible condition that can show up on your skin. This way, you'll be able to take the necessary steps to erase these unattractive signs of aging.

To help you identify the different conditions that can appear on your skin, here's a list of common factors to consider, just so you'll know what you're looking for.

➤ **Wrinkles and lines.** Creases in the skin—however deep and defined—have a variety of causes that aren't just old age. For instance, overexposure to the sun can cause dry, crêpe-like skin with anything from fine lines to deep furrows. Extreme weight loss can result in wrinkly, hanging skin. Smoking etches lines on the face, especially around the lips and eyes, and worry creases the brow.

➤ **Dermatitis and eczema.** *Dermatitis* refers to any inflammation of the skin. *Eczema* is a specific form of dermatitis, usually internally provoked by allergies. *Contact dermatitis* is a reaction to certain substances that touch the skin. This might be a plant, such as poison ivy, or a chemical, such as bleach or soap.

➤ **Psoriasis.** Scales that itch something fierce. As your skin sloughs away, new cells, produced beneath the surface, replace it. In psoriasis, cell reproduction is speeded up in some

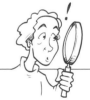

Age Alert

Damage done to the skin in childhood can haunt you as an adult. Be it frequent sunburns or untreated acne and scars, these problems persist into adulthood. It's never too early—or late—to take steps to correct them.

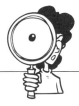

WatchWord

Lipofuscin refers to liver-colored brown markings on the skin that are commonly called age spots. They appear all over the body, especially in areas that are exposed to the sun.

areas—faster than the outermost cells can be shed. The result is deep pink, raised or thickened patches covered with white scales.

➤ **Cellulite.** Pockets of fat concentrated just under the skin that look like a grapefruit peel and feel like a bunch of hard grapes.

➤ **Age spots (*Lipofuscin*).** Often called "liver spots" because of their brown color, these unsightly discolorations mottle the skin's appearance. They are found most often on the hands, chest, and face but can show up anywhere. They have nothing to do with the liver but come from staying too long in the sun. Older skin does not tan evenly and tends to overproduce patches of pigment.

➤ **Freckles/moles.** When pigmented cells clump together, you get freckles or their larger, more colorful, cousins, moles. They can be almost any color—from pink to black—or any shape—circular, oval, and irregular. They can be flat or smooth and even hairy. Most are harmless; however, it's a good idea to have any moles checked periodically by a dermatologist to monitor any changes, which may indicate skin cancer.

➤ **Warts.** You won't get warts from kissing frogs. These "seedy" growths usually appear on the hands and bottoms of the feet. They are caused by a highly contagious virus and need to be removed by your health care practitioner, because they have a way of coming back.

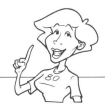

Voice of Experience

"When clients come into my salon, they are surprised that I spend more time discussing what they eat than I do telling them about skincare and cosmetics. As you wouldn't put makeup on a dirty face, you cannot cover up a lifetime of bad eating habits. This is a radically different concept from what is generally taught in the West, but believe me, it's true."

—Helen Lee, Ford model, owner of The Helen Lee Day Spa, author of *The Tao of Beauty: Chinese Herbal Secrets to Feeling Good and Looking Great* (Broadway Books, 1999)

➤ **Sun damage.** Dry, leathery skin is but one result of prolonged overexposure to the sun. Think *The Old Man and the Sea.* Increased freckling is the mildest manifestation; skin cancer, the most treacherous. Most commonly, sun-damaged skin is tanned—not as in golden brown, but as in cowhide. If you've ever lived in the Sun Belt, you know what we mean.

➤ **Scars.** These marks in the skin are memorials to the body's ability to heal. Often, these are barely visible, but sometimes they are dramatically defined, widened, or enlarged, yet remain within the boundaries of the initial injury or incision. Thicker, harder scar tissue that extends the perimeters of the initial injury is called a *keloid.* This tissue develops when the body continues to produce collagen after the wound has healed.

➤ **Surgery.** Any place where a surgical incision has been made should be noted, because the skin has been compromised in the area of the incision. Be especially conscious of any cosmetic or reconstructive operations you have had, including face-lifts, collagen injections, liposuction, etc.

➤ **Dermabrasion/skin peels.** These procedures are done to remove damage from the skin's surface. Skin that has been treated by such medical processes is left more sensitive, even delicate, and must be cared for accordingly.

➤ **Blemishes.** A rather subjective term, you might say that one woman's tiny blemish is another woman's catastrophe. For purposes of this BodyCheck, we're talking about pimples and temporary breakouts.

➤ **Adult acne.** This is a condition that should be treated medically. If you have it, you already know it's there.

➤ **Boils and carbuncles.** A *boil* is an infection of a hair follicle, usually caused by bacteria. The follicle becomes inflamed and painful as white blood cells—which collect at the site to fight the infection—along with bacteria and dead skin cells, form pus within the infected area. A *carbuncle* is either an especially large boil or a cluster of boils. Without medical intervention, boils can cause serious systemic infections.

➤ **Chapped areas.** This uncomfortable condition results from unprotected exposure to environmental conditions that take the natural moisture from your skin. This might be your lips (irritated by licking to keep them moist rather than applying a protective balm), your hands, cheeks, or anywhere your skin is exposed to harsh weather.

➤ **Oiliness.** When the oil glands in your skin become overactive, oiliness can become a problem.

➤ **Calluses and corns.** Caused by rubbing and wear and tear, calluses occur as toughened, hardened areas of skin build up to resist the abuse. Check your fingers, especially if you hold a pen too tightly or play a musical instrument, and palms if you work without gloves. Also examine your feet closely for calluses on your heels, toes, and soles. Corns are small, less than one fifth inch, while calluses are considerably larger.

➤ **Podiatric (foot) problems.** If you have problems with your feet, other than discomfort from wearing too-tight shoes, you already know what they are. Aside from calluses and corns, make note of any structural deformities of your toes, the height of your arch and instep, and the condition of your soles. Most common are *bunions*—bony protrusions from the outside edge of the joint at the base of the big toe.

➤ **Sagging skin.** Loss of muscle tone is the primary cause of sagging skin, with extreme weight loss coming in second. Correcting this age-adding condition entails targeted exercise and deep massage treatments. Surgery is a final recourse.

➤ **Enlarged pores.** Sometimes as we grow older, our skin—especially on the face—becomes coarser and our pores enlarged. They may also become clogged with pollutants, hardened body oils, and cosmetics.

➤ **Abnormal hairiness.** Any unwanted hair growth on the face, limbs, or torso can be upsetting. Although an increase in facial hair is common as a woman ages, it is not generally a cause for concern. If the hairiness appeared when you began taking a medication for seizures, birth control, or bleeding between periods, let your doctor know. If the hair growth is accompanied by an unexplained weight gain, deepening voice, and the absence of periods, you may be experiencing a hormonal disorder.

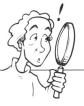

Age Alert

When you first see imperfections on your skin—especially crow's-feet and wrinkles on your face or neck—you may feel discouraged. Take heart: The reason we ask you to identify these signs of aging is that we will be giving you ways to remedy most of them. What's more important, we'll show you how to stop new imperfections from forming.

BodyCheck for Your Skin

On the following figures, mark the places where any of these conditions show up. For example, if there's a chicken-pox scar in the center of your forehead, put a dot on the appropriate spot and then write "Chicken-pox scar on forehead" in the space at the right. Mark and describe every imperfection or irregularity that you see—front and back, head to toe—until you've created a map of your skin as it looks today. Be sure to give your hands and feet a close look, too.

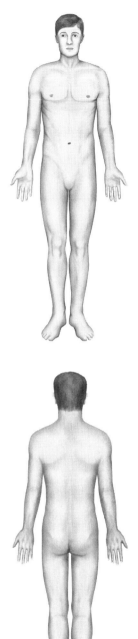

Front

_____
_____
_____
_____
_____
_____
_____
_____

Back

_____
_____
_____
_____
_____
_____
_____
_____

19

Don't Let Your Flaws Floor You

It's amazing how many unexpected irregularities crop up all over our bodies as we age. What's even more amazing is that we are prone either to overlook them or passively accept them.

We assert that you must not ignore them, nor should you accept them as inevitable signs of aging. If you allow them to take over, they will.

Later on in this book, we'll give you some powerful age-reversing tips that will restore young-looking skin.

Facing Your Feelings About Aging

At this point, you may be thinking, "I never knew there was so much wrong with my skin."

Seeing yourself in this graphic form gives you a new awareness that may stir up a stew of unexpected negative feelings. Rather than letting them discourage you, use them to motivate you to do what it takes to turn things around.

Now that you've studied the physical condition of your skin and made note of what it looks like, it's time to take stock of how you feel about it. The following exercise enables you to draw out the thoughts and opinions you hold about your skin.

Ironically, while these thoughts about our skin may appear superficial, they are, in fact, indicative of how we view ourselves. They are not limited to simple likes and dislikes of external characteristics; they color our entire self-perception. That's why it's vital to identify what we like, dislike, hate, and love about our skin.

How I Feel About My Skin

Things I ...			
Like	Dislike	Hate	Love
————	————	————	————
————	————	————	————
————	————	————	————
————	————	————	————
————	————	————	————
————	————	————	————
————	————	————	————
————	————	————	————
————	————	————	————
————	————	————	————

You *Can* Turn It Around

Here we are at the beginning of our age-reversing work, so it's expected that the columns listing things that you dislike and hate will be crowded with complaints.

In time, as you master our techniques to look and feel younger, you will notice that the balance will shift in favor of the things you like, and even love, about your skin … and about yourself.

Does Your Makeup Age You?

If your makeup style has not changed since high school, it's out-of-date. Likewise, if you share lipstick and eye-shadow shades with your 16-year-old, you may think that you look young and hip. In reality, you look weird and out of place. If you have any doubts, ask your daughter.

Before you can create a new, younger look, you'll want to take stock of every skincare and makeup product you own—not just the cosmetics you use every day. This means listing that dark foundation you picked up last September to extend last summer's tan and that sparkly body glistener you got for that big New Year's Eve party.

Make sure to check that drawer in the bathroom, as well as every handbag, makeup kit, and tote you've used in the past year, just in case you've missed something. Sniff everything, and if it doesn't smell fresh, pitch it.

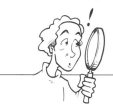

Age Alert

Remember, anything that's more than a year old should be discarded. Even the best cosmetics have a limited shelf life after they've been opened. Protect your skin and toss them out. In fact, if you can't remember when you purchased a product (especially mascara, foundation, and lipstick), throw it out, too. Bacteria can grow on that mascara wand and cause conjunctivitis and other eye problems. If you have a cold sore, the dye in your lipstick can cause infection. The lipstick itself can spread the virus.

Skincare and Makeup Inventory

Here's a checklist to guide you. List everything, even if you have more than one of something—two mascaras, three lipsticks, etc.

❏ Foundations   ❏ Eyebrow pencils

❏ Concealers   ❏ Mascaras

❏ Blush/bronzers   ❏ Lip liners

❏ Contour powders/creams   ❏ Lipsticks

❏ Eye shadows   ❏ Lip glosses

❏ Eye liners   ❏ Lip balms

- ❏ Cleansers
- ❏ Soaps
- ❏ Exfoliant/skin scrubs
- ❏ Bath oils
- ❏ Bath salts
- ❏ Masks/masques and other facial products
- ❏ Moisturizers
- ❏ Toners/after-shaves
- ❏ Shaving cream/gel
- ❏ Night cream
- ❏ Under-eye cream

- ❏ Neck and body creams
- ❏ Sunscreens
- ❏ Tanning products
- ❏ Hand lotions
- ❏ Cuticle cream
- ❏ Nail enamel/sealants, etc.
- ❏ Polish remover
- ❏ Foot creams
- ❏ Deodorants
- ❏ And anything else you couldn't resist buying

Cosmetic Cleanup

This list covers just about everything you might have accumulated to take care of and beautify your face and body. You'll begin to notice how cluttered your bathroom counter or medicine chest has become with products you rarely use.

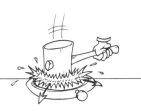

Time Stopper

Note to the guys: We know you don't wear makeup, but you do shave, shower, and clean your skin. Many items on this Skincare and Makeup Inventory pertain to you, not just to women.

How often have you purchased something that offers the promise of defying age or eternalizing youth only to discover that it doesn't deliver the goods? And what about those samples you picked up at the makeup counter? Young and beautiful forever, the clerk said.

You might be saving things because they were expensive—or because they were free—and you don't want to waste money. Ultimately, anything you're not happy using is a waste, so overcome your false economy and clean up your space.

Within a week after you've tossed them out—if that long—you'll have forgotten all about them, anyway. We call such a major cleanup a *Blitz*. Throughout the book, you'll learn how to unclutter every area of your life so you'll have room to grow younger.

Rub-a-Dub-Scrub

Bet you didn't know a lot of people don't know how to wash their faces. In fact, skincare is too often done so routinely, without a thought, that most people couldn't tell you what they do, or even what products they use, without having to think about it first.

Soap and water aren't enough. In fact, they can be aging. So, if you're going to start feeling and looking young now, you're going to have to make a few changes. And, as you know by now, change begins when we acknowledge what we're doing—right now.

How Do You Wash Your Face?

Write down your complete daily skincare routine, from the time you wake up until bedtime. Be specific. Include the products you use, and even the kinds of washcloths, towel, skin brush, razor, moisturizer, after-shave, and toner you use.

Morning:_____

Bedtime:_____

Other:_____

Skin treatments done weekly:_____

Skin treatments done monthly:_____

Now that you're completely conscious of how you care for your skin, you're ready to put in the corrections to give yourself cleaner, healthier, and younger-looking and -feeling skin.

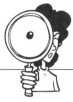

WatchWord

A **Blitz** involves going through every area of potential clutter and eliminating whatever is in your way, blocking your youth-filled future. This means actually throwing out everything you haven't used in a year—outdated cosmetics, shoes you no longer wear, clothes that don't fit ... or don't make you happy. You get the picture.

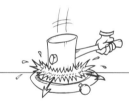

Time Stopper

Most popular commercial soaps that are advertised as great for the complexion really aren't. They are harsh for the delicate skin of the face and too drying for everywhere else.

The Least You Need to Know

➤ Early signs of aging show up on the skin.

➤ Be aware of every freckle and mole, as well as dry skin patches and callused skin. Track any changes.

➤ Confronting your feelings about how your skin is aging helps you take steps to improve it.

➤ Discard all cosmetics and skincare products that are more than a year old.

➤ Start replacing cosmetics and skincare products with those that are all-natural and cruelty-free.

➤ Skincare is not just for women. Men need special care, too.

➤ Professional facials—at least twice a year—are worth their weight in gold.

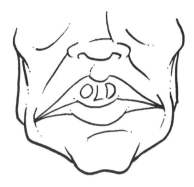

What Does Your Mouth Say About You?

Your mouth is a tattletale. The kindest, most gentle people in the world can be seen as mean-spirited if their lips are tightly pursed or their teeth yellow and jagged.

That's why you'll want to know if your mouth and teeth match the person you are. If you haven't taken care of them, your teeth and gums may have eroded and added years to your appearance and dulled your smile.

Often, as we age, we smile less—not because we're sad but because we are self-conscious about the poor condition of our teeth and gums. What a shame to be denying ourselves and the world the joy of a warm and open smile! We assure you this can be corrected with dedicated care.

By the time you've worked your way through this chapter, you will be able to present yourself to your dentist as a knowledgeable partner in the proper maintenance of your mouth. With today's innovative corrective dental procedures, you can have a beautiful mouth and smile, no matter how old you are.

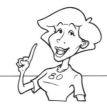

Voice of Experience

According to Dr. Gerry Herman, a top New York prosthodontist, most people think they're taking adequate care of their teeth if they brush twice a day. When Dr. Herman asked patients to demonstrate how long they brush, he realized that most people brush for only about 30 seconds. That's hardly enough to freshen the surface. He recommends that patients purchase a small timer and brush their teeth for a full two minutes. People reported that, at first, it actually felt like an eternity.

A Close-Up Look

Yes. This is the part where you will evaluate the assets and liabilities of your mouth both inside and out. You'll take a really close look at your lips, teeth, and gums. Oh, and your tongue, too.

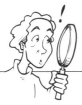

Age Alert

When you first start brushing your teeth long enough to really do some good, you may find that your gums bleed. This will disappear as soon as the condition of your gums improves from this additional stimulation.

When we started this chapter, we interviewed Dr. Gerry Herman of New York's Park 56 Dental Group to get his expert opinion on the correlation between teeth and youth. We expected him to jump right in and describe healthy teeth and gums and give us a long list of what to look for and what to do. To our surprise, he zeroed in on the lips and the areas around the mouth. We had no clue how much attention a dentist pays to the outside of the mouth even before looking at what's inside.

Dr. Herman's discussion of a truly healthy mouth and what could go wrong certainly changed our perspective. We decided to share his wisdom with you, starting with his careful description of what to look for in your own evaluation. Here goes. Place yourself before a well-lit mirror and … smile.

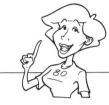

Voice of Experience

"For attractive lips, speak words of kindness."

—Audrey Hepburn

Start with Your Lips

Not everyone can boast of full and sensuous lips like those of Mick Jagger or the enormous smile of Julia Roberts, but that shouldn't stop us from having wonderful lips of our own. Large or small, lined or unlined, lips are the perfect frame for the mouth, becoming the ultimate mode of verbal—and nonverbal—expression.

The following list tells you what to look for.

Lip List

Lips:

Note the condition of your lips. Are they ...

➤ Dry or moist?

➤ Chapped or smooth?

➤ Tight or soft?

➤ Blotched or evenly colored?

➤ Pale or pink?

➤ Lined or unlined?

➤ Any lesions?

➤ Cold sores?

➤ Scars?

Area around mouth:

➤ *Nasolabial fold?*

➤ Sides of mouth?

➤ Chin?

➤ Unwanted facial hair?

➤ Jaw line?

Facial Observations

Before opening your mouth, look at your face smiling and then your face at rest. Check for symmetry, or balance, in the position and shape of your mouth. Do you like what you see?

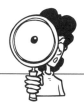

WatchWord

The **nasolabial fold** is the crease that runs between the nose and the upper lip. It adds individuality and an interesting contour to the face.

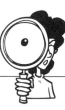

WatchWord

Located on both sides of the face, connecting the movable lower jaw—the mandible—to the stationary bones of the skull, the **temporomandibular joint** **(TMJ)** is what allows the mouth to open and close. Any dysfunction in the TMJ can cause headaches and severe neck and jaw pain, especially when opening the mouth wide. People who have this condition often hear clicking and popping sounds and frequently experience a deviation of the jaw when opening their mouths.

The Mouth in Motion

After you've observed the general condition of your mouth and lips, you'll want to check out your mouth in motion.

Eating, drinking, talking, smiling, kissing—all involve the entire face, not just the mouth. When considering the role the mouth plays in aging, it's important to get a good sense of how the rest of your face feels and looks. Also take note of your chin, as well as the flexibility of your *temporomandibular joint (TMJ)*, neck, and shoulders.

A lot of people who suffer from stress and tension are unable to open their mouths fully or have pain when opening their jaw, or the jaw deviates to one side or the other, upsetting the symmetry of the face.

We would have never guessed that the condition of the mouth and teeth depends on all these factors. It's amazing how we take so much for granted. Were it not for Dr. Herman, we never would have known how much is involved with a simple smile.

Open Wide

Now it's time to take a look at your pearly whites. Presuming, of course, they're either pearly or white at this point. We can't pretend that this isn't a bit scary. Very few aspects are quite as daunting as the loss of teeth.

Little by little, teeth become more and more of an issue as we age. We fear becoming old and toothless, remembering unappealing clicks and hisses emanating from our denture-wearing grandparents.

In this BodyCheck, you'll study the inside of your mouth like you've never seen it before. Dr. Herman provided us with a list of what to look for. As you did in Chapter 2, "How Old Does Your Skin Look?" with the Skin BodyCheck, you will mark off all the different places in which these conditions appear in and around your mouth.

We will be giving you pointers on how to correct almost all of these problems later on, but in the meanwhile, identifying them is the essential first step in creating a magnificent mouth.

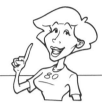

Voice of Experience

Hattie had relatively straight, attractive teeth, but over time and many cups of tea, they had turned quite yellow. Because of faulty early dental work, she also needed a bridge and an implant plus several extractions. Initially, she found this very depressing and hesitated before taking the necessary corrective actions. Since TV appearances, book signings, and lectures demanded that she radiate with a youthful, glowing smile, she had no other choice but to move ahead. Besides, Hattie loves to smile. She was not without fear when she finally decided to invest in the dental procedures that restored her winning smile. Though it took considerable work and money, she loves her teeth and hasn't had a moment's regret.

Mouth BodyCheck

Look for the following conditions and locate any on the figures that accompany this exercise.

Teeth:

Top: _____   # Bottom: _____

Color: _____   Overlapping: _____

Size: _____   Cracks in enamel: _____

Shape: _____   Chips/fractures: _____

Symmetry: _____   Surface condition: _____

Evenness: _____   Cavities: _____

Upper teeth:

Old fillings (especially darkened silver amalgams): _____

Upper teeth.

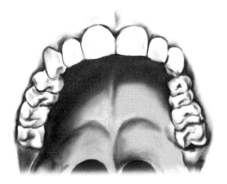

Lower teeth.

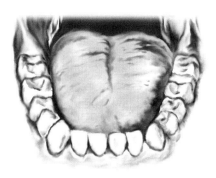

Lower teeth:

Visible plaque: ____

Stains from tobacco, coffee, and tea: ____

Missing teeth: ____

Loose teeth: ____

Caps: ____

Laminations: ____

Implants: ____

Bridgework: ____

Visible hardware from partial dentures: ____

Orthodontia:: ____

Spaces between teeth: ____

Spaces at gumline: ____

More about mouthcare:

How often do you brush your teeth?: ____

For how many minutes?: ____

How often do you floss? Rubber-tip massage?: ____

Do you stimulate your gums with a plaque remover like STIM-U-DENT?: ____
How often?: ____

Do you like what you see?: ____

How did this BodyCheck of your mouth make you feel?: ____

Getting a Grip on Gums

Here's something else to sink your teeth into: Your gums. Healthy gums are stippled and colored pink to rosy purple, depending on your complexion. They are firm and smooth, fitting snuggly against the base of the teeth. Unhealthy gums—perish the thought—are often pale and bleed easily. They are swollen and appear to be peeling away from the teeth. Receding gums allow openings between the teeth at the gumlines, creating unsightly spaces that can trap food. This allows pockets of infection to form, which can result in tooth loss.

Look at your gums with care and make notes on the figures of any conditions you see.

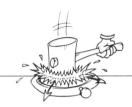

Time Stopper

If a certain condition is something you'd rather not face, it's probably one that needs facing. The sooner you take action, the sooner the rewards.

Stick Out Your Tongue and Say Ah!

Like the teeth and gums, the tongue and cheeks are vital to maintaining a youthful mouth. To complete your assessment of your mouth, we ask that you stick out your tongue and take a look.

The tongue and inner cheeks can serve as internal petrie dishes, encouraging bacterial growth and fostering illness. And because it can become coated with bacteria, food particles, even fungi and excess cells, the tongue can be a source of odor and disease.

There is no standard "normal," healthy tongue. All look different. They have all sorts of stuff on the surface and sides. The top is fuzzy, covered with *papillae* (teeny hair-like projections of tissue), surrounded by clusters of taste buds. Normally, these papillae are smooth and pink, crisscrossed by gentle fissures, which reveal the deeper red

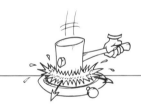

Time Stopper

Receding gums give you that long-in-the-tooth look often associated with aging. To keep your mouth looking young at any age, keep your gums strong and supple and your teeth free of tartar—a.k.a. plaque. Floss and brush daily, using a soft-bristle brush, and massage your gums regularly with a rubber tip to promote healthy circulation. If bleeding occurs, see your dentist. You probably need a deep cleaning.

muscular body of the tongue. The bottom and sides are smooth, although there may be *crenations,* or teeth marks, along the sides.

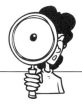

WatchWord

The *sides* of your tongue often have ridges or **crenations** that are the result of the tongue pressing against the teeth. As long as these crenations are not raw or bleeding, they present no problems.

The inner cheeks should be silky smooth and deep pink. Beware of sores and rough spots that don't heal within a week. If you happen to be a habitual cheek-biter, you'll want to break that habit. Openings in the linings in the cheek invite infection.

Odd as it may seem, the tongue happens to be the strongest muscle in the body. Unlike most of our muscles though, it doesn't move anything but itself.

We don't give much thought to our tongues, though our language makes constant allusions to it: "Hold your tongue" to quiet someone; "Tongue in cheek" to indicate sarcasm. Children enjoy tongue tricks and sounds. And we love using it when kissing.

All in all, the tongue is not a body part to be over-looked, so let's look it over now.

Tongue Test

Look for ...

Abnormal coloration—especially toward the back.

Swelling.

Fissures.

Growths/nodules.

Crenations (especially if raw).

How far you can stick it out.

How flexible it is.

How you can—or can't—curl it.

How far you can push it into each cheek.

Vein patterns under the tongue and floor of the mouth.

Open sores or tender spots.

Texture of inner cheeks.

Color of inner cheeks.

Breath Mint, Anyone?

Now you've looked over your entire mouth, both inside and out. Is your mouth exam over? No way.

There's one more factor that must be considered: bad breath.

Have you ever winced when someone came at you to kiss you and you were blown away by the smell? We've all had that experience. And we hate to tell you, it's worked both ways.

From time to time, everyone has bouts of halitosis. While bad breath, according to the old Confucius jokes, is better than no breath at all, it may make the top 10 list of repulsive body odors.

Garlic and other smelly foods are the most benign culprits to cause bad breath. They disappear within a day, presuming you've not eaten more of them.

The most persistent source of breath odor, aside from smoking, is tartar on the teeth. Accumulated bacteria make your breath smell like rotting garbage as it erodes the health of your gums. If after brushing your teeth and using a mouthwash, you still have odor, it's time for a thorough dental cleaning.

And if *that* doesn't solve your problems, you probably have a digestive disorder that must be treated. Consult your health care practitioner. Not only will that sweeten your breath, but a thorough exam also will detect conditions that may not have been spotted otherwise.

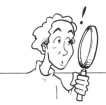

Age Alert

One of the primary sites of oral cancer is the lips. The second most common is the tongue.

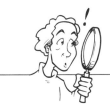

Age Alert

A toothache shows all over your body.

The Lick Trick

We don't always know how our breath smells, and it's something people hesitate to bring up lest they embarrass us or hurt our feelings. Yet we all would rather have sweet-smelling breath all the time. How can we know?

Cupping your hands over your mouth and nose and breathing into them to check your breath doesn't work, but there's one breath-check technique that really works.

If you suspect that your breath is stinky, lick your palm and smell it while it's still wet. If you don't like what you smell, you can be sure your breath is foul. The quickest remedy is to bite into, not just swallow, two capsules of BreathAsure®. That covers all the bases, handling odor in the mouth and the digestive system.

> ### The Least You Need to Know
>
> ➤ To look young, teeth and gums require attentive care.
>
> ➤ No one needs to settle for misshapen and discolored teeth.
>
> ➤ An uneven bite causes undue stress to your teeth and jaw.
>
> ➤ Nothing is more uplifting than a beautiful smile.
>
> ➤ It's essential to brush your teeth for a full two minutes at least twice a day.
>
> ➤ Bad breath is a major turnoff.

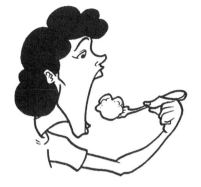

The Ins and Outs of Eating

Possibly the most notorious sign of aging—aside from gray hair and wrinkles—is "middle-aged spread."

Even if you've lived on meat and potatoes, burgers, and pizza since you were a child without gaining a spare ounce, you begin to notice that your body is changing. All of a sudden your belt is too tight and none of your pants fit. That holiday weight gain you were always able to drop in a couple of weeks by laying off desserts has taken up permanent residence. You can't imagine what's going on—you're still playing golf on weekends and even going to the gym a couple of times a week.

It's time to face facts: Your *metabolism* is slowing down and your body simply can't handle the same types and combinations of food that it once could. What once fueled your young, active body now becomes wrapped around your waist.

The good news is that this is not a terminal condition. We'll teach you how to change your diet to jump-start your metabolism and add exercises and massage techniques to help your body function efficiently.

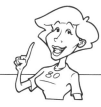

Voice of Experience

"Man is not nourished by what he swallows but by what he digests and uses."

—Hippocrates

What's on Your Plate?

If you happen to be the one in five billion who only eats fruits, vegetables, and grains, never craves desserts or pizza, and thinks chocolate bars are bricks, you can overlook this section. But if you're like almost everyone else in the world (including us), with cravings for junk food and other poor eating habits, read on and learn how proper eating makes the difference between being thin or heavy, weak or strong, young or old.

Most of us never realize that the foods we eat control the foods we eat. This statement may sound odd, but actually what it describes is a phenomenon almost everyone has experienced. We start the day with the best of intentions, resolving that we won't eat sugary desserts or stuff ourselves, and what's more, we'll exercise. In our minds, this seems entirely possible. Then what happens? We eat. And what, how, when, and why we eat controls of the rest of our day.

The fact is that certain foods, and combinations of foods, throw our systems off.

That's why it is essential to get a profile of what you eat normally in the course of a day, as well as why and when you eat, so that you'll be able to design a food plan that will leave you feeling and looking young and trim.

Keeping an Eating Diary

Before you can alter the way you eat to stay young, you need to be aware of what you are already eating

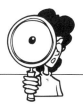

WatchWord

Your body transforms food, air, and other nutrients into a form it can use to function properly; it does this through a series of chemical processes known as **metabolism.** These functions have taken the blame for many an extra pound and have fostered a whole lot of excuses for overeating and laziness. Excuses aside, a sluggish metabolism can become a real concern as you age. It can be diagnosed easily, however, and remedied by diet and exercise changes.

on a typical day. For this evaluation, we recommend that you record your food for two days—one day during the week and one day on the weekend.

You'll notice that this is not just a food list. We've added a Reason for Eating column specifically to make you conscious of your relationship with the food you eat, and not just the food itself.

As soon as you eat anything (a meal, a snack, or those cups of coffee at work), *immediately* note the day, date, and time. Also note what and how much you ate, making sure to add the reason for eating.

Write EVERYTHING down. It's human nature to forget those lethal little snacks we indulge in when we need a boost.

The time of day may be 7 A.M., and the reason for eating may be that it's breakfast time; but then again, it could be 2 A.M., and you could be eating because you had an argument with your spouse right before you went to bed and you're still wrestling with your frustration; or it's 9 P.M., and you're sitting in front of the TV mindlessly munching popcorn after a frustrating day.

Resist the temptation to edit your diary. You're the only one who'll see it. Don't feel you have to be virtuous or feel guilty because you ate an entire pint of ice cream in one sitting. Everyone overeats from time to time—even disciplined dancers and athletes. If you ate it or drank it, write it down, even if it's embarrassing.

Fill out the three columns completely. Why you ate something is as important as what and when you ate. Pay attention to your answers in the third column, and you'll find that hunger is not always your primary motivation for eating.

Initially you may say that you are eating because it's lunchtime; however, once you look closely at your food choices, as well as how much you eat, you may discover that you are eating out of anger or frustration.

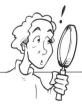

Age Alert

Tell the total truth. Don't only list foods you should have eaten or even what you intended to eat. Include everything—even that second bagel with extra cream cheese you mindlessly polished off at brunch and the bag of chips you crunched while waiting for the train. Yes—what you eat standing up or on the run counts.

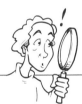

Age Alert

Brush your teeth soon after every meal. You will not only deter plaque, cavities, and gum disease, but you will also clean your palate and, consequently, be less inclined to nibble. This trick also helps chase the munchies away. If you crave a between-meal snack, pick up your toothbrush and scrub away that urge.

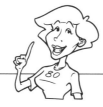

Voice of Experience

We all have heard people say they eat like a bird and then wonder why they can't lose weight. Unconscious eating is one of the most prevalent ways we gain weight. These detailed food diaries will open your eyes to what you actually eat each day. Yes, what you eat right out of the container as you stand in front of the fridge in the middle of the night does have calories and fat grams and must be included.

For example:

Sample Eating Diary, Weekday

What I Ate and How Much (# of Portions, Size)	Time of Day	Why I Ate (Activities, Circumstances)	How I Felt (Emotions, Body Sensations)
8 oz. OJ (frozen) Sesame bagel with scallion cream cheese two large coffees cream, sugar	Monday 8:45 A.M.	Breakfast; picked up at bagel shop; ate at desk while opening mail	Guilty; too much coffee but still hungry hungry; groggy

Eating Diary, Weekday

What I Ate and How Much (# of Portions, Size)	Time of Day	Why I Ate (Activities, Circumstances)	How I Felt (Emotions, Body Sensations)
_____	_____	_____	_____
_____	_____	_____	_____
_____	_____	_____	_____
_____	_____	_____	_____
_____	_____	_____	_____
_____	_____	_____	_____
_____	_____	_____	_____

What I Ate and How Much (# of Portions, Size)	Time of Day	Why I Ate (Activities, Circumstances)	How I Felt (Emotions, Body Sensations)
_____	_____	_____	_____
_____	_____	_____	_____
_____	_____	_____	_____
_____	_____	_____	_____
_____	_____	_____	_____
_____	_____	_____	_____
_____	_____	_____	_____
_____	_____	_____	_____
_____	_____	_____	_____
_____	_____	_____	_____
_____	_____	_____	_____
_____	_____	_____	_____
_____	_____	_____	_____
_____	_____	_____	_____

Eating Diary, Weekend

What I Ate and How Much (# of Portions, Size)	Time of Day	Why I Ate (Activities, Circumstances)	How I Felt (Emotions, Body Sensations)
_____	_____	_____	_____
_____	_____	_____	_____
_____	_____	_____	_____
_____	_____	_____	_____
_____	_____	_____	_____
_____	_____	_____	_____
_____	_____	_____	_____
_____	_____	_____	_____
_____	_____	_____	_____
_____	_____	_____	_____
_____	_____	_____	_____
_____	_____	_____	_____
_____	_____	_____	_____
_____	_____	_____	_____

An Eating History Lesson

You'll also want to make note of your diet habits through the years. Look back and make note of how many diets you've been on and how food makes you feel.

➤ How successful were you at losing the weight you desired?

➤ Were you able to keep it off?

➤ For how long?

➤ Do you often feel tired and sleepy after eating?

➤ Do you feel jittery after consuming caffeine and sugar?

All of this information will help you create a profile of how your body relates to food.

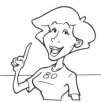

Voice of Experience

Don't panic: You won't be deprived of delicious meals—or have to eat bird-size portions. In developing my RetroAge® program, I've uncovered a wealth of delectable foods that are so super healthy you may find them sinful. So changing how you eat will be a pleasure, not a punishment.

—Hattie

The Food and Energy Connection

How your body converts the food you eat into fuel for energy—metabolism—alters with age. Part of the reason for this is that digestion becomes less efficient, making your body unable to absorb the necessary nutrients to keep it functioning at an optimal level.

You'll also notice how your energy level fluctuates during the course of a day. How you feel after eating certain foods is indicative of this process. A heavy meal of meat and potatoes usually leaves you sleepy and bloated, certainly in no shape to play ball or take a hike. Everyone has energy slumps from time to time, but these slumps should not be depleting.

If you are finding yourself drained of energy and unable to concentrate, you'll want to reexamine your eating habits. The sugary snacks and caffeine-filled drinks you take to boost your energy give you a temporary lift, only to drop you into another slump. This vicious cycle can become debilitating and fosters food addictions.

Consider how your energy levels shift during a day in creating your eating profile.

The Matter of Digestion

How your body processes the food you eat is every bit as important as the food itself, especially when we're concentrating on looking and feeling younger.

In our ongoing attempt to be thin, or fit, or young, we turn from one diet to another. First, we try an all-protein plan and lose 10 pounds. Then, when we resume eating in our "normal" way, we gain back those pounds, plus three or four more for good measure. So we go on a juice fast, which promises a 12- to 15-pound loss in a very short time. Or we adopt this month's hot new diet plan and, sure enough, we lose weight again … only to regain it as soon as we resume our regular mode of eating.

Many of us diet for years on end in search of the perfect body and boundless energy and find ourselves wondering why our weight goes up and down and we're always tired.

If we eat foods that are supposed to be good for us, why aren't we in radiant health? Why do we feel sluggish and old? What are we overlooking?

The answer to this question is DIGESTION. Most of us think of our digestive systems only if we have an upset stomach, constipation, or diarrhea.

Rather than give you an elaborate inventory to examine how well, or how poorly, your digestive system works, we'll just ask you to *observe* how you feel after eating different foods. Consider your energy levels; moods; state of alertness; and whether you feel light or heavy, sluggish, sleepy, or even ill. Keep checking your body's reactions to different foods and beverages.

The body's capacity to digest different foods changes over time. Even though you once had an ironclad stomach, you may now find that certain foods no longer agree with you. Actually, this is a blessing. This is your body's way of calling attention to the changes you need to make to stay healthy and youthful.

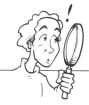

Age Alert

Even if you're not ill, your body may not be digesting food efficiently. By the time most symptoms are apparent, you can be sure that the problem has been brewing for months or even years.

With each improvement you make in your diet, you will experience an immediate shift in how you feel and look. You might want to write down your feelings so you can compare how you feel as your age-reversal moves along.

So, before we give you the tools to fine-tune your digestive system, we ask that you evaluate how your body handles food. We rarely discuss our digestive problems with anyone other than our doctor—and then, only when we're suffering.

The Process of Elimination

You can be sure we had many second thoughts about including this topic in this book. Would we offend our readers? Should we even broach the subject for fear of turning people off? Thank goodness for June Allison. Her Depend Undergarments® commercials paved the way for us to deal candidly with this highly personal subject.

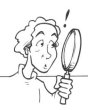

Age Alert

Unless your digestion and elimination processes are working on all cylinders, you'll be overweight and likely to age before your time.

In light of the increase in diseases of the bladder, colon, and rectum, as well as the discomfort and embarrassment of incontinence and other less-attractive conditions most often associated with aging, we decided to tackle this topic with you.

While certain aspects of aging—like gray hair and sagging muscles—are primarily aesthetic, these less-visible signs are not merely uncomfortable or unpleasant, but can be indicative of serious medical conditions that require treatment.

Once again, we ask that you take inventory of how your body eliminates its wastes. In reversing our own aging, we had to put embarrassment and reservations aside. We hope you'll do the same. Here goes …

Elimination Assessment

Ask yourself these questions so that you can be aware of what's going on with your body's capacity to eliminate waste matter and toxins through urination and bowel movements.

Urinary tract:

Frequency and ease of urination:

How many times during the day do you urinate?

Do you ever experience pain or burning when urinating?

Do you feel that you have completely emptied your bladder after urinating?

Do you experience frequent kidney, bladder, or urinary-tract infections?

How often do you get up during the night to urinate?

Do you experience *incontinence* (involuntary urination)? How often? Since when?

Do you retain fluid? Examples: Swelling of feet, ankles, hands. How often?

Do you take *diuretics* (substances or drugs that increase the discharge of urine)?

Intestines:

Frequency and ease of bowel movements:

How many bowel movements do you have per day?

Do you ever go more than one day without having a bowel movement? How many days?

Do you have to strain?

Do you experience pain?

Are you often constipated?

Do you ever find blood in your stool?

Do you ever find mucus in your stool?

Do you often have diarrhea?

Do you take laxatives?

Do you receive enemas?

Do you receive colonic irrigation treatments?

Do you experience flatulence? (Are you gassy?)

Do you feel bloated after meals?

Is your lower abdomen hard and *distended* (swelled, as if from internal pressure)?

Do you experience chronic pain in your lower abdomen?

The Connection Between Toilet Habits and Youth

We believe that the connection between toilet habits and youth has never been fully addressed. If there's one topic that everyone seeks to avoid, this is it. The butt, pun intended, of jokes and jeers, the importance of elimination can't be avoided.

How we get rid of the food we take in makes the difference between being sluggish and bloated and being vital and energized.

By thoroughly exploring everything in the questionnaire, you will know how well your body is doing its job. For one thing, it's not okay to have chronic digestive problems. In order to sell products, advertisements talk about chronic indigestion as if it's to be expected. The fact that your corner drug store is stocked with an array of remedies for these disturbances doesn't make them normal.

Time Stopper

The term "at your age" is not encouraging. In fact, it's insulting and condescending. Resist buying into that limited way of thinking. It'll destroy your dreams.

43

Unless your body is efficiently eliminating its wastes at least once a day, your metabolism will be slow, your stomach will protrude, and you'll feel out of sorts.

If there's any point we want to drive home, it's that you shouldn't accept the unacceptable. You may keep hearing, even from your doctor, that this or that condition is to be expected "at your age." We emphatically disagree.

That phrase "at your age" is a real downer. As far as we're concerned, there is no one way to age, either good or bad. This book enables you to decide how young, fit, healthy, and happy you want to be, regardless of age.

The Least You Need to Know

➤ You must be in touch with what, when, why, and how you feel when you eat.

➤ What you've eaten in the past affects your health today.

➤ Getting rid of destructive eating patterns provides immediate positive physical results, even though you will probably experience withdrawal symptoms.

➤ Plan your meals around foods that give you energy without draining you.

➤ To stay young and healthy, your digestion must function properly.

➤ Consistent elimination of toxins makes for a youthful body.

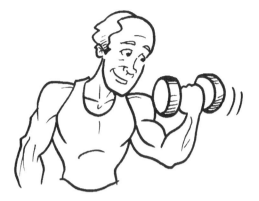

Chapter 5

A Body of Exercise

In This Chapter

➤ How fit are you right now?

➤ How fit do you want to be?

➤ The key three: aerobics, flexibility, strength

➤ Do you exercise enough?

➤ How do you feel about your body?

Certain fortunate individuals are blessed with a naturally high level of fitness, while others must battle for strength, endurance, and flexibility their entire lives.

No matter how blessed you are, if you want to age well, you're going to have to exercise *every single day*. Now this doesn't mean that you have to go to the gym or do a formal exercise regime seven days a week. It *does* mean that you must perform regular physical activity that engages all muscle groups and body parts to some degree every single day.

In the days before modern conveniences, physical activity was a natural part of each day. We didn't have to think of scheduling time with a trainer to lift weights or to take an aerobics class. Our daily chores took care of that. A walk through a supermarket is nothing when you compare it to planting and harvesting your own crops; and tossing your laundry from the washer into the dryer hardly qualifies as work when you consider what it took to stand over a wash tub and then lug everything outside to hang on a clothesline to dry.

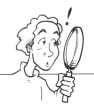

Age Alert

Regular exercise reduces your appetite, because it helps to control blood-sugar levels and leads to a steady state associated with feeling full. Aerobic exercise cuts your appetite in the short run because it raises your body temperature.

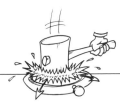

Time Stopper

At this moment, you may be a couch potato—or even a mashed potato, for that matter—but it's never too late to get moving. Studies show that people have been able to develop muscle mass even in their 80s and 90s. The more you move, the more you'll be able to move.

Also we weren't sitting in a car or on a bus to get from place to place. And we certainly weren't hanging around the house in front of the TV or computer screen. We were getting on with life, and it kept us moving.

That kept us naturally fit.

It's no big news that times have changed. And who would want to go back to those days anyway? We find ourselves in a dilemma: We've made life easier, but the very amenities that simplify our tasks have removed the need for vigorous activity. Consequently, while health advancements have made it possible for us to live longer, we are less fit than ever before. Obesity is rampant and inactivity the norm.

Assessing Your Strengths and Weaknesses

In this Exercise Profile, you will ask yourself questions about your exercise habits and level of fitness.

As you consider each question, you'll become aware of not only how much—or how little—physical activity you do in the course of a day, but also where your strengths and weaknesses lie. You may be surprised to find that some ordinary activities—such as mopping the floor, vacuuming, scrubbing the tub, and mowing the lawn—provide you with a valuable workout. And you may be shocked to find that you are exercising much less than is necessary to stay young and fit.

The Exercise Profile is divided into three parts. In the first part, you identify the specific exercises you perform to increase *aerobic* capacity, flexibility, and strength. The second part involves activities performed in the course of a day that enhance fitness, and the third addresses how your body reacts to it all.

The Three Keys

The body's condition can be gauged by three criteria: aerobic capacity, flexibility, and strength. These three components combine to create a perfectly balanced fitness regimen.

Few people, if any, are blessed equally in all three areas. A person with natural fitness generally is strong in two of these areas. That's why it is important to isolate these areas and concentrate attention on where you are least adept. Just look at a hulking linebacker: His muscles are highly developed and powerful, yet his flexibility is nil. That's why many coaches bring in ballet and yoga instructors to help their athletes loosen up and prevent injuries.

Each time Hattie goes to the Caribbean island of Anguilla to work, she is reminded by Louis Price, her massage therapist and exercise trainer, that she's been neglecting necessary strength training. Her flexibility and aerobic capacity are both terrific, but she won't keep her bones and muscles strong without strength and resistance training. Of course she balks at first, but ultimately heeds his advice once she gets home and re-enrolls at her health club.

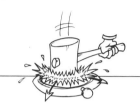

Time Stopper

Aerobic capacity, flexibility, and strength are the three key characteristics of a youthful body. Most people are weak in at least one of these areas. Identify which are your strengths and weaknesses so you can balance your body's level of fitness.

Aerobics

The word *aerobic* has been bandied about over the past decade or two—ever since Jane Fonda ordered everyone to go for the burn. Practically any exercise that involves repeated movement provides some aerobic benefit; however, for an exercise to be truly aerobic, it must elevate the heart rate for a specific amount of time relative to age and weight.

Repeated aerobic exercise improves the body's aerobic capacity. This, in turn, increases stamina as well as heart-lung capacity.

Flexibility

Flexibility refers to the body's ability to bend and stretch, lengthening the musculature easily, without strain or injury. This is certainly a hallmark of youth. If you have any doubts, just look how infants suck their toes.

This elasticity tends to lessen as we age, but exercises designed to stretch the body can restore much of what is lost.

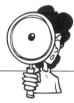

WatchWord

Simply put, **aerobic** refers to heart function. Aerobic exercise is exercise that gets your heart pumping through repeated contractions of large muscle groups against low resistance. Walking, bike riding, playing tennis or basketball, dancing, cross-country skiing, jumping rope ... all of these activities tend to burn lots of calories and, when done consistently and for enough time, contribute to weight loss.

It's particularly important to warm up your muscles before beginning any stretch work. If you don't prepare your body, you risk injury.

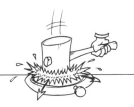

Time Stopper

Exercise in any form burns calories. Regular exercise also helps your body retain protein and minerals. It increases your heart and lung capacities, raises your metabolism, increases oxygen in your blood cells, promotes digestion, and enhances your overall stamina and muscle tone. You'll also strengthen your bones and deter the development of osteoporosis. In short, exercise is integral to total fitness.

Strength

Strength is perhaps the most obvious element in the exercise triad. Unfortunately, loss of muscle mass and weakness often go along with the aging process. At one time, such atrophy was considered normal. Recent studies repeatedly prove that this wasting away is neither inevitable nor irreversible. Muscle mass can continue to develop throughout one's entire life.

This is a perfect example of how it's never too late to reverse aging. Strength training develops muscles that are already weak from disuse and also restores bone density.

Exercise Profile

Assessing the Three Keys:

➤ **Aerobics.** How much do you do every day?

➤ **Flexibility.** What stretches do you do daily?

➤ **Strength.** What muscle-building exercises do you do daily?

Identifying Everyday Exercises:

➤ How many hours of physical activity do you get in a typical day? Include shopping, walking, climbing stairs, house and yard work, and all actions that involve concentrated movement.

➤ How many hours of formal fitness activity do you do in a day? Include the gym, jogging, sports, cycling for transportation, movement classes, and dancing.

Assessing Your Body's Response to Exercise:

➤ How do you feel after you've exercised?

➤ Are you energized, or do you feel exhausted?

➤ Do you experience dizziness or shortness of breath?

➤ Do you frequently get muscle cramps or "charley horses"?

➤ Are you awakened at night by muscle spasms?

Ranking Your Level of Fitness

➤ On a sale of 1 to 10, with 10 being Excellent, how do you rank your level of fitness?

➤ On the same scale, rank how fit you want to be.

Are You Exercising Enough?

Several books and exercise gurus assert that a half-hour of exercise every day is sufficient to keep you in shape. We emphatically disagree. Although a half-hour of structured movement is certainly better than no time at all, your body requires at least a full hour of physical activity every day to maintain optimal fitness.

This is not to say it has to be done in one 60-minute chunk, nor does it have to be a session at the gym or on the court. It can be dispersed over the course of the day.

Before you run through your litany of reasons for *not* getting in a workout (such as you're too tired to even think about it), there's plenty of evidence proving that any form of physical activity relieves sluggishness and lack of energy. Something as simple as a brisk walk around the block or a short ride on your stationary bike will do the trick.

Of course, every time you feel pooped out, you'll forget this. We do until we push past our world-class laziness—yes, we both admit to this. (How else do you think we picked up all these tips?)

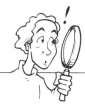

Age Alert

If you can't speak while you are exercising to increase your heart rate, you're overdoing it. Slow down. Your heart is beating too fast.

Physical Changes You Wish Hadn't Happened

Isn't it cruel of us to ask you to acknowledge areas of your body that seem to have gone to seed? We dare to tread this territory because we believe that many of the seemingly irreversible signs of aging can be erased. This is not the usual way of viewing the aging process!

Culturally, we have been conditioned to passively expect deteriorating physical stamina and loss of condition. This does not have to be. Just look at Jack LaLanne. He's just one of the earliest examples

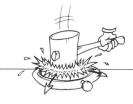

Time Stopper

Although it *can* be, exercise doesn't *have* to be boring. All you have to do is vary your program. Work out with Jane or Richard one day, go for a swim the next, ride your bicycle the third, and take long walks with a friend.

of an individual who decided that ordinary aging was not for him. More and more people are making the same choice to live a vital, physically fit, and full life, consciously making the lifestyle changes that ensure this result.

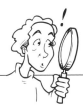

Age Alert

When setting your weight-loss goals, be realistic about how much weight you need to lose and how long it will take you to lose it. Remember: You didn't gain that extra 45 pounds overnight, or even during the past week. You certainly won't lose that weight overnight, or even in a week or 10 days.

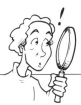

Age Alert

Hate is such a strong emotion. Yet many of us look at ourselves in the mirror with revulsion. If you can change the hate you feel about what you see to something gentler, like dislike, you'll free yourself from the paralyzing force hatred has on you.

So, once again we ask that you be honest and admit what's really bothering you about your body and its level of fitness.

How Do You See Your Body?

The Scottish poet Robert Burns wrote, "Oh would some power the Giftie gie us, to see ourselves as others see us."

In truth, most of us are unaware of how other people see us—and deep down, we don't want to know. All we want is the good stuff.

The last time we asked you to strip down and assess your body, it was for the purpose of identifying skin problems. This time, we want you to take note of how you *feel* about your body.

This time, you won't just be looking for problems. You'll take note of the "good stuff," too. Certainly, you'll be admitting the things you hate about how your body looks, but we also want you to openly acknowledge what you love about what you see.

If you're overweight, for example, you may find yourself obsessing over bulges and bumps. Instead of being bogged down in these negatives, shift your awareness to your face or your hands. Focus on your good points, whatever and wherever they may be.

Nature has provided us with a fascinating balance. Very rarely does one person embody all great traits. Nor does one person register only negatives. There's a plus here, a minus there ... and plenty of neutrals to round out the mix.

In making this assessment, be rigorously honest, but don't be cruel to yourself. By the time you've finished this exercise, you may be surprised at how much there is to love about your body. Yes, even with its myriad flaws.

How I Feel About My Body

Stand before a full-length mirror and write down what you see before you. If you don't feel brave enough to do this naked, go ahead and do it with clothes on.

Things I hate about my body:

_____

_____

_____

_____

Things I dislike:

_____

_____

_____

_____

Things I like:

_____

_____

_____

_____

Things I love:

_____

_____

_____

_____

What I want to change:

_____

_____

_____

_____

What I plan to do about them:

_____

_____

_____

_____

Dealing with Feelings

If you've completed these exercises with diligence, you're probably experiencing a swirl of emotional "stuff" you might prefer to ignore. Our best advice to you is *don't*.

If you're riddled with guilt over all those broken promises to exercise regularly, we ask that you be gentle with yourself. You might find it helpful to record these emotions in a journal so that you'll find the support you need when you get to Part 3, "Looking and Feeling Young with E.A.S.E.," where we introduce an E.A.S.E. (pronounced *EASY*) program of Exercise, Attitude, Skincare, and Eating.

The Least You Need to Know

➤ Everyday chores can be turned into exercise.

➤ Exercise must become an "always" thing.

➤ The more you exercise, the more you'll be able to exercise.

➤ Aging doesn't mean weakness.

➤ Learning to love your body helps you look and feel younger—and much happier.

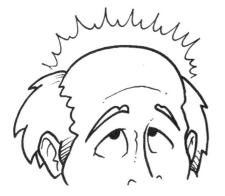

Chapter 6

Is Your Hair Your Crowning Glory?

In This Chapter

➤ How hair defines our identity

➤ Hair loss and aging

➤ How to look at your hair

➤ The health of your scalp

➤ What your hairstyle says about you

➤ Hair and scalp BodyCheck

We are often identified by our hair—especially by its color and style. The little girl who had a little curl, right in the middle of her forehead. The Blonde Bombshell. The guy with the red hair and freckles. The girl with the frizzy brown hair. In fact, hair is perhaps our most identifying feature, even more than skin, eye color, and body type.

For most of our lives, we awaken wondering if it's going to be a good hair day or a bad one. We gauge how attractive we are by the appearance of our hair. To assure that we measure up, we are ever mindful of the latest celebrity looks on television and in magazines, comparing our own hair to the locks in the media. We clip photos of these stars from *People* magazine to show the person who styles our humble head and pray that, miraculously, we'll measure up. (Women take note: Guys do this, too … only they're not so obvious about it.)

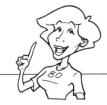

Voice of Experience

Colin Lively, color director of Elizabeth Arden's flagship Fifth Avenue salon in New York City, contends that hairstylists and customers speak two different languages. "I've spent many hours with crying clients who say, 'I didn't get what I asked for. I told her I wanted the same style as _____ ...' (some celebrity ... Madonna, Whitney Houston, Sophia Loren). And I've spent equal hours with crying stylists who say, 'But I gave her exactly what she said she wanted.'"

Colin, who owned salons in Cleveland, Ohio, for 15 years before making the move to New York, advises that such miscommunication is to be expected when both client and stylist have unrealistic expectations about what one visit can do. "It takes at least three visits—a cut plus two trims—before you both feel 100 percent satisfied."

Then, when we hit our 30s, our awareness shifts from style to color and quantity. How many gray hairs sprouted overnight? How much is left on our heads or on the comb; how much washed down the drain?

By the time men reach 40, they are wondering if there will be any hair left to fret about at all. This worry is intensified if their maternal grandfathers and uncles are bald, since the gene that spurs hair loss is passed along by the mother.

A Little Loss

Everyone loses a little hair every day—80 to 100 strands is normal. In times of extreme stress or illness, we may experience severe hair loss. When hair falls out but the bulb is still alive, hair can grow back—often more luxuriantly than before. Once the root is gone, though, no new hair can grow.

While women don't generally have serious hair loss, many experience thinning after childbirth and menopause, when their estrogen levels drop. The one exception is the disease *alopecia areata,* which can affect both genders. Pattern baldness, on the other hand, occurs only in men.

The good news is that, for most people, severe hair loss is not an inevitability of aging.

Balding is predominant among Caucasians. In other races, it appears to be a consequence of civilization—refined foods, pollutants, stress, and illness—rather than age.

Hair loss may occur as we age, but there are numerous ways to handle this condition. Some are quite simple and reasonably priced, while others, such as surgical hair-replacement procedures, are complex and costly. Once administered by prescription only, topical medications that stimulate hair regrowth—such as Rogaine—have been proven effective in many cases and are now sold over the counter.

What *Is* Hair, Anyway?

As humans, we have some type of fuzz all over our bodies—except for the palms of our hands, the soles of our feet, and hmmm, our lips. For the purposes of this chapter, the only hair we're going to talk about is the hair on our heads.

A healthy strand of hair is smooth, from root to tip. It should have extreme tensile strength, so you can pull it tightly without breaking it. It grows about half an inch a month for two to four years before it is shed.

Hair is 97 percent protein, with the remaining 3 percent made up of amino acids, minerals, and assorted trace elements. This explains why what we eat is so critical to the health of our hair and scalp.

Like your skin, hair is a reflection of your physical well-being. As a rule, dull, brittle, lifeless hair is indicative of some degree of illness, while shining, elastic hair signifies good health.

Damage Control

Both hair and scalp can be traumatized by external influences. Perming and straightening chemicals, bleaching and dying, sprays and other styling products, as well as harsh shampoos can do serious damage.

Watch out for excessive blow drying, especially at high temperatures, which literally burns the hair

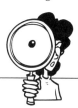

WatchWord

Unlike balding that occurs naturally as a receding hairline or patch at the crown, **alopecia areata** is a specific disease that can result in anything from round, bald patches to total hair loss all over the body. Sometimes, alopecia-caused balding stops within a few months, and can be treated medically with steroids. The cause of alopecia is unknown and can affect anyone at any age. In fact, most people who will develop alopecia do so before their 30s.

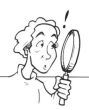

Age Alert

Just as sun can damage the skin in other areas of the body, it can damage the scalp. This can impede hair growth—one more reason to wear a hat any time you're out in the sun.

and scalp. Pollution, sun, and even extreme cold also ravage the delicate structure of each strand.

When Grandma was a girl, she washed her hair no more than once a week, if that often, using the same lye-based cake of soap that she used for her laundry. She brushed it a hundred strokes every night and every morning pinned it up in a tight knot. Grandpa tamed his hair with grease and water and always wore a hat.

Oh, how things have changed. With today's airborne pollutants, holes in the earth's ozone layer, high-fat foods, steam heat, hot rollers, and blow dryers, daily washing with a shampoo formulated to restore balance to hair and scalp is almost a necessity.

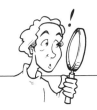

Age Alert

Dull, out-of-condition hair, especially when wet, is prone to tangling. Yanking those knots out with a brush only makes them worse. Slowly and carefully work them out with a wide-toothed, nonmetal comb.

Products to care for and style our hair are common in the daily grooming process of women *and* men, regardless of age. You may be surprised to find how many products—from shampoos and conditioners, to styling gels and sprays, even treatments for dryness and medicines for dandruff—are on the market to control damage.

When shopping for hair care products, the most expensive are not necessarily the most effective. Too often, the cost of packaging and advertising accounts for the high price.

Read the ingredients and avoid products with isopropyl alcohol; sodium laurel sulfate; and various red, yellow, and blue dyes—all of which have been implicated in causing cancer.

Start at the Root

The hair root, or bulb, is embedded about $1/8$- to $1/5$-inch into the scalp, with its intricate maze of nerves and sebaceous (oil) glands. It is fed by a network of blood vessels that provide nutrients necessary for growth. Although hair has no feeling, it is not dead. It receives a blood supply but has no nerve connections of its own to provide sensation.

Pull a hair from your head and look closely. You should be able to see a tiny, rounded knot—the bulb-like root—around the hair where it grows from the scalp.

A healthy root is twice the size of the hair shaft. If it's not, or if it's pointed, the root is weak or possibly dead. You may want to check a hair from another part of your head to see if the weakness was just in that single hair or whether it appears elsewhere.

How hair grows.

(Illustration by Shari Deoki)

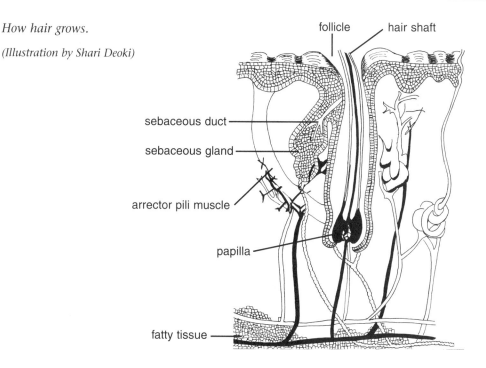

follicle   hair shaft

sebaceous duct

sebaceous gland

arrector pili muscle

papilla

fatty tissue

When examining the root of your hair, the next best thing to an electron microscope is a 100-watt light bulb and a piece of white paper. Place the hair on the paper and examine it under the bright, unshaded light bulb. You'll be able to see the shape of the root as well as its color.

This same technique will allow you to see the density and texture of the hair itself, too.

Scalped!

A healthy scalp provides a strong foundation for a splendid head of hair. When it is too dry or too oily, problems can occur:

➤ A dry, itchy scalp may signify *dandruff*, a mild form of eczema. More unsightly than unhealthy, this flaking is, as a rule, easily treated with medicated shampoos and scalp massage.

➤ If excessive oiliness is present, the *sebaceous glands* of the scalp are overactive. The waxy oil these glands produce not only gives hair a greasy appearance but also builds up on the scalp. When *sebum* hardens, it blocks blood flow, starving the roots embedded in the scalp. The result: hair loss.

Excess oil also makes your head a "dirt magnet," giving it the appearance of a string mop.

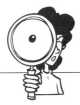

WatchWord

The **sebaceous glands** are tiny glands embedded in the skin that produce a waxy substance—**sebum**—that helps keep the skin's surface supple and prevents it from drying out. When the glands in the scalp are overproductive, hair has an oily appearance. When the buildup of sebum hardens, blood flow through the scalp is slowed, which weakens hair at the root.

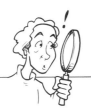

Age Alert

There are hundreds of external preparations designed to enhance the appearance of hair and improve its condition. Certainly, what you use on your hair can make a huge difference; however, as with your skin, the best treatment we can give our hair and scalp is a balanced, healthy diet. Hair needs nourishment from within. Every day is a bad hair day if your eating habits are poor.

➤ To test whether your scalp is abnormally oily, part your hair at the crown and blot your scalp with a white tissue. If any residue shows, you have an oily scalp. While you're at it, sniff the tissue. If it doesn't smell sweet and clean, wash your hair pronto.

➤ To determine whether it's unduly dry, part your hair in a place near the crown where you can see it. Run a fine-tooth comb gently across the scalp, and check to see how much flaking you pick up.

Is Your Hairdo a Don't?

Hairstyle, like cosmetics and clothing, can nail your age in a flash. If you're sporting the same color, length, and style you did when you finished school, it's time to break free of that time warp. A style that worked when you were young probably won't be flattering today.

While it may seem wise to find a look that suits you and stick with it, you're probably dating yourself. This is especially true if you've been wearing it exactly the same way for as little as five years. It might be flattering, but is it exciting?

Why then are there men who still sweep and spray their hair into the disco 'do they wore to the prom? Probably for the same reason there are women who still have the same Farrah cut they've worn since graduation: It's safe.

Women who just pull their hair back into a loose ponytail and guys who tell their barbers to "take a little off the top" are running in the same slow lane.

We recommend that you put safety aside and get adventuresome. The results may thrill you.

If you enjoy your current cut and style but suspect there's still something dated about how you look, get a color consultation. A color change just might do the trick. If you're not sure if a complete change of color would make the difference, try a demi- or semi-permanent color. Permanent colors last for months and require retouching every four to six weeks, while demi-permanent color shampoos in and lasts for six to eight *weeks*. Semi-permanent color is gone within six to eight *washings*. And if you really hate a color, you can wash your hair every day and get rid of it in little more than a week. This way, you can experiment with something new and chic without making a long-term commitment.

When Hattie's hair started turning gray, she very much enjoyed the novelty of her shining, newly silvered tresses. After several years, she decided to soften the look and find out for herself if blondes really do have more fun. For the next eight years, she had a ball as a blonde. In the course of developing her age-reversing program, *RetroAge®,* her feelings about herself as an "older woman" shifted so radically that she chose to stop dying her hair. She enjoys the distinction of being a beautiful woman "of a certain age" with radiant platinum hair. It certainly gets a lot of attention … which she thoroughly enjoys. In fact, inspired by this very book, Hattie cut off her shoulder-length locks that you see pictured in the exercises and has updated her look with a short, sassy style.

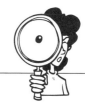

WatchWord

Hattie trademarked and registered the word **RetroAge** to introduce a paradigm shift in the way we view aging. She hopes it will become part of the English language to bring consciousness to the possibility of aging in reverse. It will appear in the dictionary as a verb: *RetroAge* (v.t.) the act of aging in reverse.

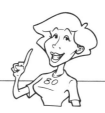

Voice of Experience

"Like so many other professions, hairstylists have become specialists," advises Elizabeth Arden's color director Colin Lively. He cautions, "There are so many changes going on in color and styling techniques that it's rare for one person to be skilled in both areas. Some haircutters are talented colorists and vice versa, but to make sure you're getting the best care in each department, look for someone who specializes in one or the other."

When it comes to hair color and cut, throw caution to the wind and get adventuresome. A savvy stylist will be able to bring your look up to date while taking years off your age. Change may feel scary at first, but part of staying young is constant change.

Hair is a great place to start.

The great thing about hair is that, even if you're dissatisfied, it will always grow back and you can try something new.

It's possible that there isn't a woman alive who hasn't wished that she had someone else's hair. Of course, we women tend to do this with every part of our body. Hair, however, does seem to get the lion's share of this attention.

When you answer these questions, also consider what you've always wished for. As you pay attention to the condition of your hair and scalp, you will be ready to design a hair look to create a new, younger you.

BodyCheck for Your Hair and Scalp

➤ Is your hair naturally straight, curly, or wavy?

➤ Do you wish it were different? In what ways?

➤ Is it fine or coarse? Thick or thin?

➤ Do you have significant hair loss? Where?

➤ Are you worried about losing your hair or balding?

➤ What is the condition of your hair? Dry, normal, oily?

➤ Is it shiny and healthy? Dull and limp?

➤ What is the condition of your scalp? Dry, normal, oily?

➤ What color was your hair when you were a child?

➤ What is the natural color of your hair now?

➤ Do you wish it were different?

➤ Do you dye your hair?

➤ At home or in a salon?

➤ What kind of color do you use? Permanent, single process, double process, demi-permanent, semi-permanent, henna?

➤ Do you perm or straighten your hair?

➤ Do you like the results?

➤ What is the length of your hair?

➤ Are you happy with this length?

➤ Is it layered or a blunt cut?

➤ Does your hairstyle flatter your face?

➤ Is it easy to take care of?

➤ How often do you wash your hair in a week?

➤ What products do you use to style your hair every day?

➤ How long does it take you to style your hair every day?

➤ How long have you worn your hair in this current style?

➤ Does your hairstyle make you feel attractive?

➤ If not, do you plan to do anything about it? By when?

To do the final part of this BodyCheck, pluck a hair from your head and look at it closely under a bright light. It works best to place the hair on a piece of paper so that you can see it clearly. Use a magnifying glass if you have one. Look at the shape of the root and the condition of the hair shaft.

As every one of us knows, our hair can be our worst or best feature. One thing's for sure—it's the part we give the most attention. Our bodies can be camouflaged in flattering clothing. We can become brilliant conversationalists, have interesting careers, develop fabulous friendships, yet the one thing that always seems to take priority is hair.

It doesn't matter whether we think this is a good idea or not—hair does have a mind of its own.

The Least You Need to Know

➤ The condition of your hair is a reflection of your health.

➤ The most expensive hair products aren't necessarily the best.

➤ The hairstyle of your youth may not be youthful today.

➤ If your hair color and style aren't contributing to a youthful look, a good hairdresser can work miracles.

➤ Hair can be your best or worst feature.

Part 2
Taking a Look at Youth

In the hubbub swirling toward the millennium, a TV commercial featured black-and-white images of a teacher in front of a late-1950s classroom of fourth- or fifth-graders saying "In the year 2000, do you know how old you will be? Can anyone do the math? You'll be my age."

A boy and girl toward the back of the classroom roll their eyes at one another in horror. Then the screen bursts into color with, presumably, the same boy and girl now grown up, bedazzled by the sights of Epcot and Disney World unfolding before them.

The obvious message Disney wants to convey is that its theme park will make you feel like a kid again. This it accomplishes convincingly. However, what stuck in our minds was the sight of those two children, horrified at the prospect of being as old as their teacher.

When we were 9 or 10, we never imagined we would be as old as our parents and teachers. We lived in the moment and enjoyed ourselves without thought of growing old. They were the grownups and we were the children, and that's how it would always be. Now we are the grownups, and we are still haunted by these early thoughts that it's really yucky to be old.

In Part 1, we asked you to get in touch with the state of your body by posing questions and looking closely at every wrinkle, ache, and change. Now, in Part 2, we begin to tell you how to use this newfound awareness so that you can start the process of looking and feeling younger. You'll learn how to use the power of your mind to alter any counterproductive feelings about aging; how to create an environment that supports your quest for youth, and exciting ways to update your appearance to reflect the new you.

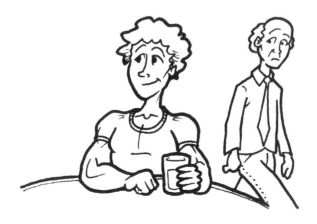

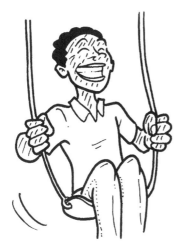

Chapter 7

Young Is as
Young Thinks

In This Chapter

➤ How you viewed aging when you were young

➤ Facing your own negative ideas about aging

➤ Facing society's negative ideas about aging

➤ Creating new attitudes about "being old"

Each of us has formed a body of beliefs about what old age is all about. These ideas, born in childhood, follow us through our entire lives, coloring our beliefs and affecting our actions. In short, our earliest perceptions exert a profound influence on our present and our future.

In this chapter, you delve into your feelings and thoughts about aging. These observations serve to help you understand exactly what youth means to you—with both its pluses and its minuses. By carefully examining your feelings, you can more effectively begin a lifelong quest for eternal youth.

For us, "eternal youth" is not a Utopian fantasy in which everyone stays 21 forever. Nor do we mean that we will be exempt from the effects of time. No one is.

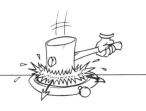

Time Stopper

Don't expect your attitudes toward aging—and yourself—to change overnight. Rome wasn't destroyed in a day.

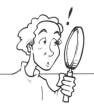

Age Alert

"We grow too soon old, and too late smart."

—Amish proverb

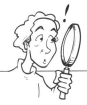

Age Alert

What you think about aging is based on your past. It may be entirely off the mark and ready for major revision, both culturally and personally. Start releasing these past-based preconceptions now.

Aging is inevitable; the image of old age in our nightmares is not. Not only can we adapt our diets and exercise routines to prolong our physical well-being, we can also initiate changes in how we *think* to create an attractive, youth-filled future. As a wise person once said, "If I'm not willing to let go of my past, my past will become my future."

Eternal youth, as we see it, is that state of mind that keeps us forever experimenting, growing, changing. Young is as young thinks.

This does not mean that we give mental imagery and thoughts of staying young precedence over action. Far from it. We must do all we can to remain physically youthful, regardless of the dates on our birth certificates. We have found that an attitude that fosters change and growth gives us the foundation from which to take the necessary actions to make sure that our bodies keep up with this attitude.

When You Were a Child

Age is a strange concept to small children. They start by grasping the differences between "little" and "big"—they are little; Mama and Daddy are big. Time is not a factor. Everything is now.

The distinctions "young" and "old" come later, as their contact with the world expands. They are young, Mom and Dad are grownups, and Grandma and Grandpa are old. Really old. Time becomes a factor, and they begin to make plans for when they become grownups.

The thought that they will someday be old is never in the picture. As they see it, they will never be old, nor do they want to be.

While being grown up is desirable, being old clearly is not. Consciously or not, we carry this message with us from childhood into adulthood. We may know, intellectually, that this is incorrect, but nothing can stop the nagging thought that being old is tantamount to being dead, or at least suspended between life and death.

What were your fantasies when you were a child? Recall your "when I grow up" dreams. Do your adult choices match these childhood wishes?

"I Don't Wanna Be Old Like Grandma!"

Your earliest impressions of what old age looks like probably came from being around your grandparents. You watched their every move and mannerism, and perhaps heard their complaints about creaking joints and assorted aches and pains. You saw them reach for their reading glasses and touch-ed their often dry, wrinkled skin. You played special games, taking care that you didn't get too rough or run too fast, because they couldn't keep up.

That children dearly love their grandparents doesn't change the fact that they don't aspire to *look* like them. There are, of course, examples of grandparents whose style and achievements inspire their grandchildren with indelible optimism about aging. But this is rare.

Think back on the impact your own grandparents imprinted on your developing consciousness. If they were not present during your early childhood, were there others, beside your parents, who shaped your beliefs? There may have been a sweet neighbor who baked cookies and spun tales about growing up on a farm. And the grandmotherly lady who led story hours at the library, transporting you to magical places far away.

Not all such influences engendered warmth—there were also the grouchy neighbor who kept every ball that bounced into his yard, or the eccentric spinster sisters who called the police at Halloween because you were making too much noise as you and your friends went door to door shouting, "Trick-or-treat!"

While fond memories of cookies and fairy tales sweeten our thoughts of the elderly, the predominant images are of wrinkled faces and shuffled steps.

You swore this would never happen to you. Did it?

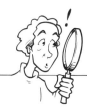

Age Alert

Fear of growing old haunts us from childhood. Some people see themselves as old at 30; others at 40 ... and over the hill at 50. We also know people in their 60s and older who are filled with energy and life. The difference between these two groups is in their attitudes. If we believe that the years we live bring inevitable changes in our minds and bodies and these changes result in old age, we age in that image. If we want to remain young as long as we live, we have to reject these traditional beliefs about time and age.

Images of Aging

Even when you watched television or went to the movies, the images of older people reflected many of these same unwanted characteristics—cranky, crotchety, and mean.

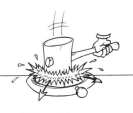

Time Stopper

Don't be afraid to express the really negative stuff. If you were afraid to visit an aging aunt because she always smelled like linament and insisted on hugging you, say so. Acknowledge your belief that all old people smell funny, and write it down. Get down and dirty without censoring your thoughts. Facing the so-called "ugly stuff" honestly will help you transform not just the way you think but the way you act as well.

The Wicked Witch of the West. Ebenezer Scrooge. These unappealing characters quickly overpowered the sweet thoughts associated with Grandma and Gramps, forging prejudices that may remain with you even today.

To begin transforming your ideas about aging, it is vital that you reconnect with your earliest thoughts. Try to recall the words you associated with aging. If adjectives such as *feeble, slow, eccentric, odd, sexless, silly, frail, absent-minded, smelly, ugly,* and *pathetic* come to mind, it's no big surprise. Those are the images we have inherited. Now's the time to get rid of them.

When you fill in the chart called "My Beliefs About Aging," you will tap your innermost beliefs about growing old. This list isn't about how you feel about your own aging. It's about how you view aging in general.

While we ask that you list only five negative ideas, you probably are carrying around many more—five will do for now, though. The second part asks that you list five good things about aging. Considering how we've been programmed, finding these plusses may be more difficult than it sounds. As you progress through this guide, the balance will make a major shift. It did for us.

My Beliefs About Aging

List five negative beliefs you have about aging:

1. _____
2. _____
3. _____
4. _____
5. _____

Now list five positive beliefs you have about aging:

1. _____
2. _____
3. _____
4. _____
5. _____

What Society Says About Aging

Baby boomers who are feverishly rebelling against the effects of time as they enter into their 50s have created a wide and affluent market for products that either guarantee youth or correct problems associated with aging.

In response, Madison Avenue has flooded the media with advertisements touting the success of these products—makeup that puts the youthful glow back in a woman's skin, medications that restore male sexual function, vitamins that increase memory and energy levels.

Not long ago, topics such as menopause and impotence were taboo. Today they are discussed openly and often in intense detail. Talk shows that never would have touched these matters now expound on intimate details without embarrassment or hesitation. When else in history could a former senator and presidential candidate confess his sexual dysfunction on national TV?

Does all this attention indicate that our collective consciousness about aging has changed? Regrettably, it has not. We may be talking more about growing older, but underlying all this rhetoric are the same fears and concerns that plagued our parents.

Beautifully photographed scenes of mature couples strolling romantically on a beach or an "older" mom playing with her toddler may give the impression that aging is acceptable, but we're still a long way from loving the aging process.

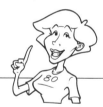

Voice of Experience

This from Hattie: "When I realized that I was going to keep aging, no matter how hard I worked to stop it, I decided that I'd better learn to love it. As soon as I quit resisting what was happening and learned to honor myself as an older woman, I became more youthful. What a shock. I can't say it's always been easy, but loving the journey has turned it into an exciting adventure."

Turning Things Around

Our aim in this book is to put a stop to this debilitating way of viewing aging once and for all. We must counter all preconceptions that an older person is no longer agile (physically or mentally), sexually vital, or even competent to carry on a worthwhile existence.

As you follow this program, you will alter your habits and your thoughts and emerge as living proof that aging can be a glorious adventure. This is the only way to eradicate society's corrosive force of *ageism*.

Self-Fulfilling Prophesy

If you expect that your body will inevitably deteriorate, your mind dull, and your sex drive diminish, it probably will happen.

Thoughts are very powerful. They have the strength to create reality, for better or worse. So doesn't it follow that the most rewarding course of action would be to concentrate your energies on creating a healthy body, an alert mind, and a fulfilling sex life?

Remember this formula:

Transformed Thinking = Transformed Aging

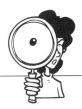

WatchWord

Ageism is a prejudiced way of viewing aging, resulting in discrimination against all people of a certain age, regardless of their abilities.

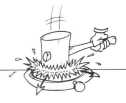

Time Stopper

You can't control time, but you can control your thoughts. Say "no" to negative thinking.

Psychologist Dr. John Kildahl, co-author of *Beyond Negative Thinking*, notes that anyone in the habit of thinking negatively will, in time, become a victim of these thoughts:

For instance, women who are in the habit of thinking negatively, that is dwelling on the things they have lost, may concentrate on menopause, the empty nest syndrome, or unfulfilled ambitions. They may feel a loss that their child-bearing years are over and that there will be a decline in sexual fervor and frequency.

He continues …

At any age, if one focuses on the parts of life that are missing, or are in danger of being lost, that person will be more apt to be discouraged and anxious, and possibly even more prone to psychosomatic illnesses.

On the other hand, healthy thinking means the person realizes that many significant life tasks have been accomplished, and that they have reached the point where they are likely to be respected and admired as a mature adult. Being recognized as someone whose opinions and actions are worthy of respect because of the experience that life has taught gives meaning to life.

People who focus on loss and limitations will age sooner than those who stay in the moment and think positively. Such negative thinking saps your strength, reduces enthusiasm, and turns life into misery.

New Attitudes for Old

Who hasn't heard the adage "You are what you think"? It's a question of attitude. Whenever your mind delivers a negative aging idea, get in the habit of turning it around immediately. If you hear the thought "You're over the hill," counter it with "I'll keep climbing, so I'll never be over the hill." The more you do this, the more efficient you'll become at stilling this destructive voice.

Yes, it is within your power to control the discouraging effect this voice can have on your life. Start doing it now.

By the time we reach our forties and fifties, we know ourselves pretty well. We cease pursuing many things that are meaningless or transitory. We stop chasing rainbows, and we look for the satisfying elements in our lives. This is not to say we have no dreams, but that we have a new, fulfilling perspective on life.

Says Dr. Kildahl …

> *Research on happiness shows that friendship with family and friends is the single most important element in happiness. Second in importance for most people is productive work. Not necessarily work that is done nine to five, but activities that provide a sense of accomplishment, and an awareness that one is making a difference in the world.*

This cannot occur if we are stewing in a vat of negativity.

Not that you need to be reminded, but here's a batch of clichés about aging that we've been hearing for years, along with the kinds of thinking that will turn them around. We call this *the flip*. By reframing a negative stereotype into an affirmative personal image, we plant the seeds of positive thinking that can alter our lives.

Cliché:	Aging makes you weak and fragile.
Flip:	I'm healthy and strong enough to do what pleases me.
Cliché:	Old people are prone to injury.
Flip:	I work out all the time, and because of that, I'm much less susceptible to injury. My weight training helps stop bone loss and osteoporosis.
Cliché:	Old people heal slowly.
Flip:	I take such good care of my body that my immune system is terrific.
Cliché:	Older people should behave in a mature manner.
Flip:	I'll behave in any way that feels authentic to me.

Cliché:	When you are old, you should slow down and take it easy.
Flip:	I love sports and dancing and will continue to enjoy them for my entire life.
Cliché:	You've worked all your life. It's time to retire.
Flip:	I love what I do, and I have no interest in retiring.
Cliché:	Old people worry a lot.
Flip:	Time has taught me to trust my judgment and also to surrender to the power of the universe. I no longer worry about things I can't control like I did when I was young.
Cliché:	You're too old to enjoy sex.
Flip:	Sex keeps getting better for me as I learn to treasure life more and more.

The truth is, to grow old is easy; to grow young takes work. We'll have to unlearn many things we've learned. We'll need to reprogram our minds to discard the belief that time causes aging. We can replace this with an entirely new way of thinking: that time has no power in and of itself to make us old.

Once we learn to accept this at gut level, we can begin to grow younger, not just in our bodies but in our hearts and souls as well.

The Least You Need to Know

➤ Our feelings and thoughts about aging are rooted in past prejudices.

➤ Society's views have controlled our perceptions so that we fear and despise aging.

➤ You can flip negative clichés about aging into life-affirming attitudes.

➤ Transforming your thinking transforms your aging.

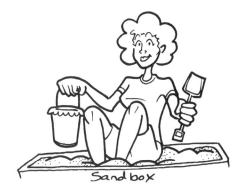

Sandbox

Chapter 8

Living in Youthful Surroundings

In This Chapter

➤ Looking at your home with fresh eyes

➤ Refreshing, renewing, and renovating your space

➤ Getting help from friends and experts

➤ Being inspired by your surroundings

➤ Eliminating toxins

Why is it that we can walk into one room and immediately feel right at home and then go into another and feel out of sorts?

Dark-colored walls and heavy upholstered furniture may cause one person to feel closed in and weighed down. Another may get a sense of warmth and stability in the same surroundings. This second person may be put on edge by the light wood tones, natural fibers, and wide expanses of glass that delight the first person's fancy.

So, as you see, it's all in the eye—and the experience—of the beholder.

Are You at Home at Home?

How we furnish our homes is an intensely personal thing, yet many of us live with things that no longer match who we are today. These might be that couch given to us by a relative who was moving to Florida, a spindly rocking chair that could use repair, that dinette set purchased at a flea market when you furnished your first apartment.

We may have consciously chosen these pieces at one point, but now, for the life of us, we can't imagine why. Do we throw them out or give them away? No. And there they stay, staring us in the face, possibly even gathering dust.

Now is a good time to consider weeding them out.

Seeing Your Surroundings with Fresh Eyes

You may be living in a home with a design and decor that hasn't changed in 20 years. The problem is, you're not the same person you were 20 years ago.

Change is the key to renewal.

When you decide to update your surroundings to support your quest to look and feel younger, you're going to be throwing away a lot of the things you've been living with for years.

The decor in your house, from the carpets on your floors to the pictures on your walls and everything in between, is there for a reason. These items are very personal and often have deep meaning for you.

It won't be easy to just toss them. But that may be exactly what you'll need to do.

Reasons vs. Excuses

Let's not fool ourselves. There are many valid reasons why you would hesitate to throw everything away and start over again, not the least being economic. Refurnishing and refurbishing can be costly. You also may have sentimental considerations; items can hold cherished memories. Many of these sentimental items you may decide to keep, and that's appropriate.

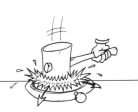

Time Stopper

A rule of thumb when deciding to keep or toss something in your home: If you wouldn't buy it if you saw it today, you really don't want it.

We don't suggest that you get rid of everything old or worn. We do, however, want you to take a hard look at what you're keeping and why.

Question your motives. Are you holding on to something because your mom gave it to you and you were too embarrassed to tell her you didn't like it? Or is it that you hate shopping? These are excuses, not reasons.

Reasons have validity, while excuses rationalize our inactivity. Inactivity keeps us old. A *reason* for not discarding a stained, worn couch is that you're saving to buy the one you love. An *excuse* for keeping it is that it's good enough ... besides, a new one will just get dirty. Can you see how this kind of thinking keeps you stuck in your past?

Just look at everything you own like you are seeing it for the very first time. Then choose to keep it, toss it, or move it.

Time for Change

Changing your environment is a radical move, but so is the decision to live a life filled with youth.

We certainly don't advocate going back to the mattress-on-the-floor and sheets-for-curtains decor of your post-college years. God forbid! A youthful environment must be one that supports the vitality and energy of the person you are today and who you expect to be in the future.

You'll have to define what this means for you. A youthful environment is different for different people. The common element is that it involves clearing away the old and bringing in the new.

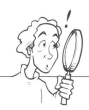

Age Alert

Clinging to possessions from your past keeps you from moving into your youth–filled future. Your mind and your photo album are great places to archive your memories. Don't clutter your living space with them.

Be Like Sherlock Holmes

When you think of updating your environment, be merciless. Zone in on every specific element, however insignificant it seems. To do this, you'll have to inspect every nook and cranny.

It's almost like dusting with a Q-tip.

What Serves You Now?

A good idea is to get a notebook to make notes as you move through your home. Be scrupulous.

In addition to the obvious signs of wear and tear, make note of things you've been putting up with. This might be that avocado-colored refrigerator, circa 1960, that clashes with everything else in your kitchen, and the table you've had since college with all the water rings and scratches. While they serve a purpose, you'd be happier if you replaced them.

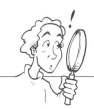

Age Alert

Rodents, roaches, and dust mites thrive in an environment filled with paper and clutter. Keep cleaning and clearing your space.

Making Your List

List what you need to replace (a light-switch plate in the living room) or repair (loose tiles around the bathtub). You might also have a wish list of things you've always wanted but have hesitated to buy.

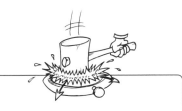

Time Stopper

To determine whether you need a paint job, just lift a picture off the wall. If you can see the silhouette of the frame, it's time to repaint. Use this as an opportunity to try out a new color or wall-covering technique.

Leave plenty of space for notes. This is not a project you will accomplish in one afternoon. The more you look, the more you'll see. You look at your home every day, so you're numb to its flaws. Your walls may be in serious need of repainting, but you can't see it until you lift a picture off the wall.

Don't Go It Alone

Most of us can't be completely objective about something as close and personal as our homes. If you know you can't trust yourself to be as critical as you need to be to get the job done, call in a friend. Ask for their honest input.

According to Joshua Wiener, owner of New York's prestigious Silverlining Interiors, this is tricky territory:

What friend would be ready to say, "Yuck, I hate that sofa, and that rug belongs in your doghouse"? It's not likely. A good friend would not want to hurt your feelings. So if you want to hear it straight, you've got to promise your friend immunity.

Call In the Experts

Even with the help of your friend, you may still have questions. "So that your home doesn't remind you of where you were or your lack of willpower to change your life, call in a decorator or architect to help you," advises Silverlining's Wiener.

He adds …

A consultation doesn't cost all that much, and you don't have to commit to using them for the entire job. There are people who hire professionals to do everything, from soup to nuts. One client who spends most of his time in Australia hired designer Eve Robinson to do his New York apartment, right down to the toothbrushes.

We add: You don't have to go that far, unless of course you want to.

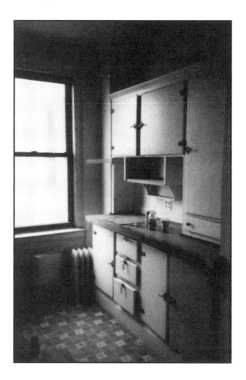

Before.

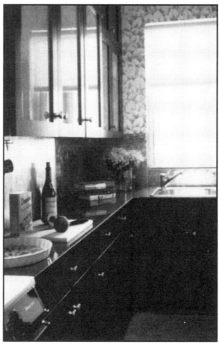

Windowed cabinets, durable countertops, and contemporary appliances and plumbing fixtures transform an out-dated kitchen into a warm, yet completely utilitarian, work space.

(Photos courtesy of Silverlining Interiors)

A Professional's Advice

We called on Ms. Robinson, whose work has been featured in *House Beautiful* and *The New York Times,* for her suggestions. She offered several valuable guidelines:

➤ Select items because you love them in your space. Always remember that you'll be living with them for some time.

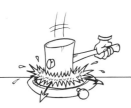

➤ Be eclectic. Choose pieces that are timeless, not all from the same time period.

➤ Get rid of excess clutter—books you'll never read again, those you plan to read but probably won't, children's toys after they've outgrown them, etc.

➤ Go through your dishes, silverware, and linens and eliminate everything you don't routinely use or don't love.

➤ Be charitable. Contribute what's cluttering your space to the Salvation Army or your favorite charity.

Time Stopper

Don't just dump everything you don't want into the garbage. Give it to a thrift shop or charity. It may be clutter to you, but it could enhance someone else's life. Besides, knowing that it's serving a useful function can overcome your reluctance to blitz.

These tips apply to redecorating your home regardless of your age; however, since this time your focus is on youth, concentrate on courageously eliminating anything that binds you to the past. Choose colors, lines, and styles that challenge your imagination. Don't be afraid to experiment. Be daring.

Blitzing Room to Room

Remember the word "Blitz" we introduced in Chapter 2, "How Old Does Your Skin Look?" It bears repeating, this time relating to your home environment:

A *Blitz* involves going through every area of potential clutter and eliminating whatever is in your way, blocking your youth-filled future.

Starting with the entrance to your home, you will want to take your notebook, a big box of heavy-duty garbage bags, several heavy cartons, and plenty of courage as you work your way from room to room.

Fill the garbage bags with things you're throwing out and the boxes with items you're giving away. Make quick decisions about what you're going to keep and what you're discarding. If you have to think too long about it, it's probably not a keeper.

Immediately move those bags and boxes out of your space. If you don't, you may be tempted to reclaim things you've already decided to get rid of. A dangerous idea.

Be Inspired by Your Home

It doesn't have to cost a fortune to have a warm, comfortable home that nurtures and inspires you. What's key is to surround yourself with a few well-chosen, meaningful personal objects that please you.

If your home is cluttered with vestiges of your past, you'll never be able to move out from under them. They keep aging, and so do you.

Make Room for the Future

As your tastes change over time, be willing to let go of the treasures of your past and make room for possibilities for your future.

Don't be concerned that you've thrown out too much. Empty space doesn't have to be thought of as a negative, but offers us an opportunity to fill it with something new, energizing, and refreshing.

Look to the East

Within the past decade, Americans have gravitated toward a centuries-old Chinese practice known as *feng shui* for advice in arranging their homes and workspaces.

This ancient art of placement determines not just where furnishings should be positioned in a house, but also where the house is built and where it faces on the lot. "The result is a home infused with loving energy," according to Shawne Mitchell, who teaches people how to nurture their spirits through her company, Soul Style. "This energy can be found in the objects that have special meaning to us, making it essential that the possessions we use to decorate our homes have special, empowering meaning for us .... The happiest people in the world are those with abundant love in their lives and in their homes."

Ms. Mitchell, who writes the "Home as Sanctuary" column for *Healthy Resorts and Spas* magazine, incorporates the practice of feng shui in her work as a consultant and realtor.

Time Stopper

You can enhance the healthfulness of both your bed and bedroom environment by paying attention to everything from the right sheets to the presence of a tropical plant or two. One hundred percent cotton sheets absorb perspiration, buckwheat husk pillows offer support, leafy plants provide oxygen, full-spectrum lighting promotes overall health, aromatherapy candles trigger relaxation, and the right color choices create the right atmosphere.

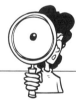

WatchWord

The ancient Chinese art of placement is known as **feng shui.** It is used to determine the arrangement of furnishings and accessories to encourage a maximum flow of energy, known as **chi,** and to create ultimate harmony.

Stay Naturally Young

If you can bring nature indoors, you will stay in touch with the youthful spirit of the environment.

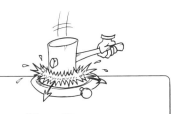

Time Stopper

Refreshment of your home environment replenishes the spirit and keeps you young.

You might be inspired by an assortment of fresh flowers or a basket of African violets bursting with blooms. A tabletop fountain that splashes water across a mound of pebbles can calm even the most jangled nerves.

A window that opens onto a park or sunset vista will give a room the illusion of space and a warmth not found when it faces a solid brick wall.

Decorators often use plants as a design element when furnishing homes. Plants offer not only their beauty, but a unique health benefit. With photosynthesis, plants use carbon dioxide, which isn't healthy for humans, and transform it into life-supporting oxygen.

Before.

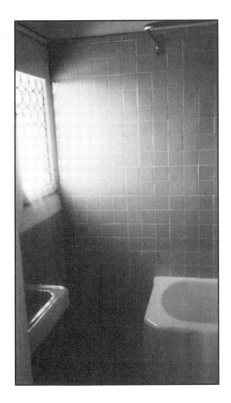

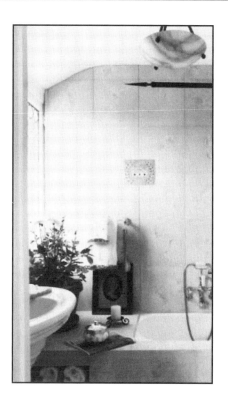

You don't need to do a major remodel to transform your aged bathroom into a luxurious bath chamber. Dated ceramic tiles in a 1950s green are replaced with 12-inch marble-like squares. Build an open cabinet to hold rolled towels at the end of the tub, creating a shelf for candles and plants, and, in place of the chipped porcelain sink, install a graceful free-standing pedestal sink.

(Photos courtesy of Silverlining Interiors)

Other natural elements, such as a tabletop display of seashells, bonsais, or an aquarium with brightly colored fish, are also sources of energy and beauty.

Even Artificial Light Can Be Healthy

Natural light is divided into colors that affect our mood and energy flow. The human eye receives light that ranges from 400 to 700 nanometers. When the days get shorter and darker in the winter, or when no sunlight enters your space, full-spectrum light can be replicated by special light bulbs.

Extensive research shows that full-spectrum light not only illuminates but also duplicates the benefits of natural daylight. Because of the balance of color provided by these light bulbs, they are glare-free, reduce eye stress, and improve concentration.

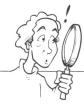

Age Alert

Wherever possible, resist using halogen light bulbs that shine directly on you. First of all, they are a potential fire hazard; more seriously, the tremendous heat they generate can be dangerous to your skin and eyes. If you do use halogen bulbs, make sure they are covered by a grid to keep anything from touching them, and that they are sufficiently filtered to protect you from their rays.

When you use full-spectrum light bulbs, you get the same quality of light as the sun ... minus the sunburn, of course. And, as a bonus, this type of light is flattering to the complexion.

Detox Your Environment

Just as you wouldn't drink polluted water, why should you live in toxic surroundings? You certainly wouldn't willingly expose yourself to asbestos or lead-based paints any more than you would inhale chemical fumes.

To live a long, youthful life, you must take steps to rid your environment—especially your home and workspace—of all potentially hazardous materials.

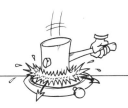

Time Stopper

Use leafy green plants to improve the air quality in your home. They're natural air purifiers, especially the non-flowering varieties that produce no pollen.

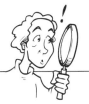

Age Alert

Whenever possible, use only environmentally safe paints, finishes, and floor finishes, as well as cleaning products. With increased consciousness of pollutants and poisons, manufacturers are now offering toxin-free products.

While you may have no control over the materials used to construct your home or the heating and air conditioning systems, you can take some simple steps to rid your environment of some of these dangers:

➤ Don't store pesticides, herbicides, fungicides, and fertilizers that you use in your garden. Seek out nontoxic garden chemicals whenever possible.

➤ Beware of fumes from paints and thinners, lacquers, floor finishes—anything that could vaporize and seep into your house. Never store these items in your attached garage or basement or inside your house.

➤ Avoid most commercial cleansers. They are filled with toxins. Purchase environmentally safe cleaning agents. Formerly available only at health food stores, these agents are becoming generally available.

➤ Avoid all products that contain ammonia or isopropyl alcohol. Very toxic.

➤ Get rid of all aluminum cookware. It's been implicated in Alzheimer's disease and other ailments.

➤ Minimize moisture in your basement and attic. Seal off exterior walls. This dampness can cultivate the growth of mold spores, which are carried through your home by a forced-air heating system.

➤ Avoid using microwave ovens whenever possible. Don't stand within eight feet of them when in use. And better yet, keep them unplugged when not in use.

➤ To keep radiation levels down, keep anything electrical—including your TV—unplugged when not in use.

The Least You Need to Know

➤ Confronting your clutter makes room for a youth-filled future.

➤ Consulting experts helps you see your home in a new perspective.

➤ Elements of nature bring fresh energy into your surroundings.

➤ Feng shui imparts inspiration and peace to your home.

➤ Full-spectrum lighting enhances your mood and your health.

➤ Toxins that contaminate your living space must be eliminated.

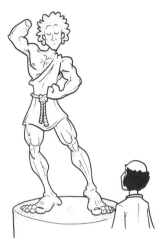

Chapter 9

Timeless Beauty

In This Chapter

➤ Learning how looks contribute to our self-image

➤ Understanding the self–image/self–esteem connection

➤ Discovering what happens to our self-image as we age

➤ Choosing a new look for a new you

➤ Bringing your hairstyle and color up to date

➤ Dealing with hair loss

There is substantial documentation that good-looking people get most of the breaks. Pretty little girls and cute little boys quickly learn to get to the head of the class with a smile. From then on, their self-esteem grows, so that by the time they're adults, they are blessed with poise and confidence.

We cannot deny that how we feel about ourselves as people is directly linked to how attractive we perceive ourselves to be—or more exactly, how we believe *others* perceive us.

The Self-Image/Self-Esteem Connection

Studies have shown that people who are regarded as physically good-looking have a higher degree of self-esteem than those who consider themselves ordinary-looking.

A person may have been an extraordinary parent, made important contributions to the community, and achieved professional and personal success and *still* be plagued by feelings of inadequacy. Too often we establish our sense of self-worth by how physically attractive we perceive ourselves to be. This self-deprecating way of thinking devalues the essence of our being.

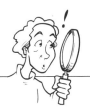

Age Alert

A word of caution: Avoid wearing perfumes, colognes, or scented lotions when you will be exposed to the sun. These products, as well as such medications as antibiotics, birth control pills, and hormone supplements, can cause blotching.

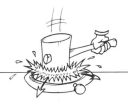

Time Stopper

Whenever you begin to put yourself down or feel discouraged about aging, it's time to take control of your negative inner voice and flip it into powerful, positive affirmations to enhance your self-esteem.

The force of negativity, be it from external sources or internal voices, can be destructive if not countered. Once again, we can flip these distorted, negative thoughts into powerful, self-affirming statements that must become second nature. Only then can their hold on us be released.

Must Self-Image Suffer as We Age?

All it takes is a sprinkling of gray hair or a couple of crow's-feet, and we're off to the races. In no time at all, we're obsessed with becoming old. We ponder our lost youth and bemoan what we envision as a rapid decline into old age.

What a strange phenomenon: Many people who once considered themselves attractive and vibrant when they were young become terrified that they will soon become old and old-looking. Often this shift in self-image is triggered by a birthday—the fortieth, for many.

Worrying About Your Lost Youth?

When the mind decides that all is lost, if you're not careful, hopelessness takes over. And with the loss of hope, one's attractiveness does suffer. It becomes a vicious circle.

Time for a Change

If you want to alter your way of being, you must actively choose to alter the way you think. As soon as you find yourself resigned to aging unattractively, it's time for a change of perspective.

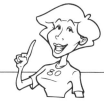

Voice of Experience

Psychologist Dr. John Kildahl tells of visiting a retirement center where there were portraits of five residents, all over the age of 100. "There was enormous dignity and beauty in the faces of those people. I stood and looked at them for a long time admiring their faces as I would admire a beautiful sculpture .... The fact that people can do something about their appearance imparts a healthier and more optimistic outlook on life."

Use the Flip technique introduced in Chapter 7, "Young Is as Young Thinks," to consciously flip your thoughts from the negative—which obviously is disempowering—to a more powerful and positive mindset.

Keep at it. Change won't happen overnight. Negative thoughts visit us throughout our entire lives. In time, however, this shift will be reflected not only in your attitude but in your physical appearance as well.

Thoughts Come First

Research indicates that thinking precedes feeling. What people think definitely determines how they feel. It is important to realize that, by changing your thoughts, you can change your feelings.

What's the mindset that you have to change? It's the one where that nagging little voice tells you that you no longer look good because you're getting old. But it doesn't stop there. It torments you with the thought that you can never be attractive again. If you listen to it long enough, you'll lose hope and quit caring for yourself.

What happens then? The nasty little voice wins.

Nobody wants that to happen, so every time you hear it, immediately counter it with a quick Flip. Repeat your positive affirmations as often as necessary to silence it. Hattie has a sentence that she repeats over and over again whenever she feels depressed: "I will not suffer; I will be happy." Sometimes she has to say it dozens of times before her sadness lifts. It works.

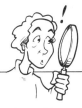

Age Alert

If your haircut and color haven't changed in years, you look older than you should. This same rule of thumb applies to makeup. Update your look by consulting professionals in the beauty biz. They'll see you with fresh eyes and advise you on how to bring your look into the present. P.S.: You don't have to purchase every product they recommend in order to benefit from their ideas.

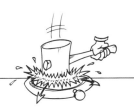

Time Stopper

Change can be threatening, or it can be exciting. Learn to enjoy the effort it takes to implement changes. You'll be doubly blessed: first with the changes themselves, and then with the pleasure of making them happen.

Finding Beauty at Every Age

As you age, your appearance undoubtedly changes. At every stage, your face and body mature, just as you lost your baby face when you reached your teens. Unless you can accept that there is beauty at every age, you fall victim to the lie that only the young are beautiful or handsome or even worthwhile.

We'll be giving you a powerful technique to enhance your self-esteem in Chapter 13, "A = ATTITUDES That Keep You Young."

Honor Yourself

In our culture, we are not taught to appreciate our appearance as we mature. This, too, must change, as it robs us of so much joy.

To honor ourselves, regardless of age, is a skill we must cultivate. Sadly, it does not come naturally.

Let's master this skill by learning to appreciate and savor ourselves as we are now.

Choosing a New Look for a New You

When we speak about honoring yourself as you are right now, we don't mean you should passively accept the effects of aging. On the contrary, looking and feeling younger is a proactive process that continues for the rest of your life. It requires constant updating and change.

You don't have to be resigned to the toll time takes on your body. It's important, however, to confront how you have aged and what bothers you about it.

Initially, admitting what displeases you might make you feel inadequate. But it is essential. It gives you direct access to what needs changing in order to update your look. Once you know where you need improvement, you will be able to formulate a plan for these changes.

Makeup Makeovers

It's astonishing how many women in their 40s, and older, are *still* applying their makeup the same way they have since … at least since their early 20s. This cosmetic time warp is guaranteed to keep you looking older than your age! Here're some pointers that will keep you looking youthful at any age:

➤ The skin around your eyes and nose is thin and readily shows red and blue tones. Apply concealer before using foundation to equalize skin color.

➤ Go for yellow-based concealers and foundations to neutralize blue and red undertones. They blend beautifully into every skin color—including Asian and African American.

➤ Pick a concealer that is a shade lighter than your skin. If it blends perfectly—like a foundation—it won't conceal anything.

➤ Use foundations formulated especially for your skin type (oily, dry, normal, combination). If you don't know what you need, ask.

➤ Make sure that your skin is thoroughly moisturized. Dry skin emphasizes wrinkles and aging.

➤ Keep experimenting until you find your best colors. The best way to test foundation is on your cheek—not on the back of your wrist or top of your hand. If at all possible, stand as close to a window as you can and match the bottle color to your cheek in natural light.

➤ Avoid sparkly blushers and eye shadows. Leave those for the kids.

➤ Pick eye shadows that contrast or complement your eye color and complexion. If your shadow color is too close to your eye color, the effect will be too blah. The colors cancel each other out.

➤ Apply mascara lightly and separate your lashes with the tip of your mascara wand for a wide-eyed look.

➤ Use either black or dark brown mascara. Save the blaring designer colors for costume parties.

➤ Set your makeup with translucent powder or one that matches your foundation.

➤ Remember: As you age, where makeup is concerned, less really is more.

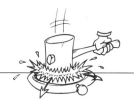

Time Stopper

Regardless of what you've heard, beauty is *never* just skin deep. True beauty radiates from within. We all possess it, but first we must claim it.

Before. 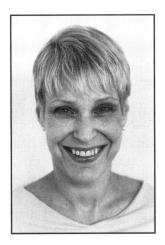 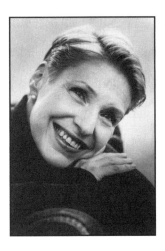 After.

An attractive woman in her early 50s, Madeleine Kaplan consulted New York makeup artist Richard Downs for advice about updating her look. Richard first evened her complexion by applying concealer over the dark circles under her eyes. Using an ivory foundation to give her face a warm glow, Richard then applied blush lightly to the "apple" of her cheeks to brighten Madeleine's smile. He used a soft taupe shadow sparingly over her eyes and applied a light touch of dark brown mascara to her lashes. He used lip liner and gloss in the same shade of coral, defining his model's lips without stark contrasting colors. Further updating Madeleine's look, Richard parted her short-cropped hair high on one side and, using gel lightly for lift, blew her hair back from her face. The look is contemporary and smart ... youthful without being too young.

(Makeup by Richard Downs; photos by Ron Catarsy)

Updating Your Hair

Contrary to what we might think at any given time, the primary purpose of the hair on our heads is not to drive us nuts. Its sole purpose is to protect our scalps from the elements. Nothing more.

On the surface, this sounds simple enough. But hair has taken on entirely new meanings, not the least being to keep us looking young.

Without the right cut, style, and products to control that willful growth, we are setting ourselves up for one bad hair day after another.

A New 'Do for You?

We don't know about you, but we don't always want our hair to look the same way every day. After all, we don't do the same thing day in and day out. We may spend our workdays chained to a computer or racing from meeting to meeting from dawn to dusk and then spend our weekends on the beach. We need to be able to adjust our hairstyles to our lifestyles.

We want options. We want to be able to choose how we wear our hair, rather than succumb to the whims of our hair. Nobody wants to look in the mirror and ask, "Well, Hair, what are you going to do today?"

Just as we don't want to wear our hair the same way every day, we also don't want to look the same way year after year.

While it can be smart to find a cut that suits you and stay with it, this practice can date you. It also limits your sense of adventure, preventing you from exploring new options.

Ask the person who cuts and styles your hair for ideas. Your stylist may be as tired of doing the same thing over and over and over as you are of looking at it.

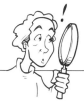

Age Alert

Even if you've found a great style and have been wearing it for years, don't hesitate to explore making changes. We may think that a style defines us, when in fact it dates us.

Different or Dramatic?

Sometimes subtle changes can bring a classic cut right up to date. A bit of layering through the crown can add softness or even height; feathering about the face can add movement.

Your stylist will know how to adapt your basic, classic cut so that it looks fresher and younger.

After trying a few simple changes, you may find that you're ready for something completely different. If you've worn your hair in a blunt cut at the shoulders for as long as you can remember, have it cut. Straight hair: Why not a perm?

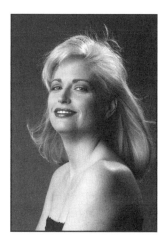 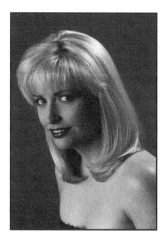

A versatile hairstyle can take you from morning to night. Blow hair out over a curved brush so that it falls about your face, or, using a light gel for control, move hair off your face.

(Photos by Susan Johann; courtesy of Colin Lively)

Hairstyling techniques and products are always being improved, so chemical processing—be it curling or coloring—is far safer than it was 10, even 5, years ago.

Besides, hair grows back.

Colorist Colin Lively paints highlights into hair to create movement and depth. This is not a home-coloring project to be taken lightly. Consult a pro so that your hair will look young ... and kissed by the sun.

(Photos by Susan Johann, courtesy of Colin Lively)

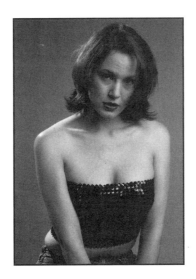 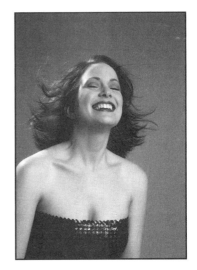

Color Changes

Long before we spot our first gray hair, our hair starts looking dull and drab. If you're adventuresome and want to bring youth back into your hair, you can always change your color.

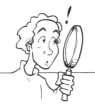

Age Alert

Just as it's important to protect your skin and eyes from the sun, it's vital to wear a hat to protect your scalp from burning and your hair from drying. For men in particular, sunscreen is not enough.

By our early 20s, our hair has lost most of its secondary tones—those shimmering highlights of our childhood. That in itself is enough to drive many women to "reach for the bleach" and color their hair years before it's time to cover any gray.

Such a pre-gray color change is called "fashion color." If your hair is light, you may want to brighten the prevailing gold or silver tone. If your hair is dark and you want enhancement rather than change, you might elect to add gold or red highlights. You may even decide to make a dramatic change and go for a different color altogether.

The addition of color can lift your spirits while keeping your hair as young-looking as you feel.

A Mane Event

The hair-and-beauty industry estimates that 80 percent of American women color their hair at one time or another. If you've never tried it, give it a thought.

Hair color is a rather subjective, and consequently confusing, matter. That's why we interviewed an expert in the field: Colin Lively, color director at New York's Elizabeth Arden Red Door Salon and Spa.

Rather than dividing hair into blonde, red, or brunette, Colin makes hair color very simple to understand. He separates it into two very specific categories: light and dark. "After all, blonde can be pale gold, almost white, or the color of an Easter chicken, and brown hair can range from a mousy tan to rich mahogany," he explains. "Light is light and dark is dark. You can't get subjective about that."

Making the Color Commitment

Whether you use color to brighten your hair or to cover gray, you'll want to decide how much you are willing to commit to the process. This is not a decision to be taken lightly. A lot of work goes into maintaining colored hair.

The three basic types of hair-coloring products vary in how long they last:

➤ *Permanent* color is used to color hair that is 50 percent gray or to provide a radical color change. You must retouch the roots every four to six weeks, depending on how fast your hair grows and its natural color. This is especially important if you've made a dramatic color change. Be sure to apply new color only to the new growth, because it could seriously damage previously dyed hair.

➤ *Demi-permanent* color covers moderate graying and gives life to dull, listless hair. These products require no bleaching to strip the pigment from the hair shaft. You shampoo them in, and they last from six to eight weeks. You can create dazzling highlights with bright or contrasting colors, because the light, gray hair provides a different base for the color than your darker, untreated hair.

➤ *Semi-permanent* color, like demi-permanent, covers gray and adds zip to dull hair. The difference is that it washes out in six to eight shampoos. This is a great way to experiment with a new hair color without risk. If you don't like the way a color looks, just keep washing until you're back where you started.

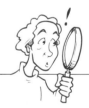

Age Alert

The more you change your hair from its natural state, the more you will have to do to keep it looking and feeling healthy. This is especially true if your hair has been given a major color change. Talk to your stylist. Color mishaps take a full year to grow out completely; bad perms take even longer.

Handle with Care

Once hair has been chemically treated by coloring, curling, or straightening, it must be treated with care:

➤ Never, ever brush wet hair. Always use a comb with rounded teeth.

➤ Always use the lowest temperature possible when blowing hair dry.

➤ Use steam rollers rather than hot rollers and curling irons.

➤ If perming colored hair, make certain that your stylist uses chemicals formulated for colored and treated hair.

➤ Buy hair care and styling products made for use on colored and treated hair. It's worth the investment.

Dealing with Hair Loss

Serious hair loss is not just a male issue. Women can also experience this problem.

This loss occurs in a variety of ways. Most commonly in men, this is a receding hairline—hereditary male pattern baldness or *androgenic alopecia*. This condition afflicts approximately half of the male population by the age of 50. It is also the cause of the overall thinning experienced by women as they age.

Geneticists contend that hair loss is a secondary sexual characteristic of males, influenced by hormones. In the case of women, stress is the predominant determinant.

Hair follicles can also be asphyxiated by the buildup of sebum, which clogs the pores of the scalp.

Alternative Measures

While medical advancements have been made to treat balding, many of these treatments are potentially hazardous to the health. Some people use these preparations, which are taken internally or applied topically, despite the risk, however. To them, balding is not an option.

If you've tried stimulating the circulation of the blood through the scalp to nourish hair at the root, thorough cleaning of the scalp and hair, and holistic and herbal treatments without success, you may want to consider a cosmetic alternative—especially wigs and hairpieces, if these appeal to you. You might also consult a qualified plastic surgeon to discuss hair implants and scalp reduction.

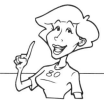

Voice of Experience

Robert Green Ingersoll, addressing the Twentieth Anniversary Dinner of the Lotos Club in 1890: "You have talked so much of old age and gray hairs and thin locks, so much about the past, that I feel sad. Now, I want to destroy the impression that baldness is a sign of age. The very youngest people I ever saw were bald."

Loving Yourself, Bald and All

Though few would consciously choose being bald as an option, accepting ourselves, whether we have hair or not, is one more opportunity for us to honor and respect ourselves for the people we've become.

The Least You Need to Know

➤ Enjoying the challenge of change keeps you looking and feeling young.

➤ When you alter your attitudes about aging, you become more attractive.

➤ Feeling good about how you *look* makes you feel good about who you *are.*

➤ Updating your makeup, haircut, and color gives your looks and your spirits a major boost.

➤ Medical, cosmetic, and psychological ways to deal with hair loss are available.

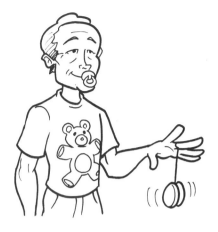

Chapter 10

Dressing for Your New Age

In This Chapter

➤ Choosing between fashion and style

➤ What your wardrobe says about you

➤ Defining an ageless look

➤ Creating a young look of your own

➤ Wardrobe blitz

The clothing we wear says a lot about us. And, since we only have one chance to make a first impression, let's make it a good one.

What we choose to wear influences how people see us. Within moments, they've made numerous decisions about who we are: accessible or cold, dated or youthful, stodgy or warm, well-off or broke … or simply suffering from bad taste. All that at a glance.

That's why it's helpful to know what your clothes say about you.

Is It Fashion or Style?

Designers and magazines have a lot to say about what's fashionable and what's not. The only trouble is that this season's fashions may not be "in" next year. Fashion, you see, is defined by prevailing attitudes and imagery and, as a result, must be in a state of constant change.

After all, fashion is a business, and business is about urging people to spend money. If fashions didn't change with each season, manufacturers would have nothing new to sell. A whole industry would go kaput.

Thankfully, this is not about to happen. Fashion is fun, and nobody wants it to disappear.

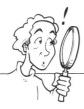

Fashion Is Fickle, Style Is Sustaining

Style, on the other hand, is quite different. It may or may not have anything to do with fashion trends. In fact, some of the most stylish people in the world wear the same kinds of clothes season after season, year after year, even decade after decade.

Most truly stylish individuals simply don't care if they're in fashion or not. They're confident about who they are and have made decisions about how they will present themselves in keeping with these personal choices.

And, surprisingly, by being true to their personal style, these people often set the tone for what's fashionable for the rest of us.

Age Alert

Before investing a lot of money in something that is the latest fashion, consider whether you'll enjoy wearing it for several years. You may like it so much that you'll buy it no matter what. Just admit that you're making a fashion choice, not necessarily a choice for long-range style.

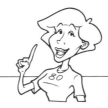

Voice of Experience

Accessories designer Priscilla Averbuck offers this bit of advice: "Your attitude is the most important thing in looking young and dressing properly. If you have the right attitude, you can pull anything off."

It's Your Choice: Conventional or Personal

We all have our cultural uniforms—the gray flannel suit if you're in advertising, navy pinstripes with a red tie if you're a banker. While women are given a few style concessions—a strand of pearls in place of a tie—and a wider spectrum of colors, these guidelines, both spoken and unspoken, dictate what's acceptable in the workplace.

There are also preconceptions about how people—especially "older people"—should dress and behave. Where is it written that a person must stop wearing bright colors or short, sexy skirts ... or bikinis ... once they reach a certain age?

If you try to recapture your lost youth by wearing clothing designed for teens, you'll miss the mark. In fact, trendy youth-culture clothing serves to emphasize your age. Beware: You risk looking foolish and out of place.

Why go backward when there are so many flattering fashions out there to choose from? Nowadays, you never have to feel limited to dowdy, dated attire. Thankfully, designers are catching on and are answering our demand for upbeat, contemporary clothing that supports our young-hearted lifestyle.

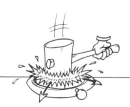

Time Stopper

When creating your personal style, make sure that you aren't bound by the stereotypes that society imposes. Dress to suit your spirit and the person you want to show to the world.

Let Your Personality Show

Without breaking from the ranks, people still manage to express their individuality regardless of age or career. They refuse to be pigeonholed by stereotypes and inject their personal choices into prevailing standards.

You've seen people who stand out in a crowd. Nothing flashy or bizarre, just distinctly personal—a special piece of jewelry, a creatively tied scarf, a fresh flower worn every day. It might be in their color choices and even in the length of their skirts and the cut of their trousers.

We know of a schoolteacher in suburban New York who dresses quite conservatively on the job. Nevertheless, every day he delights his students and colleagues with a dazzling splash of color from his collection of outrageous neckties. This is how he shows his individuality, and it works. It also keeps him young and alive, along with everyone around him.

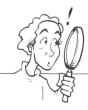

Age Alert

If you wear the same clothing year after year without adding several new elements, you'll look dated, no matter how flattering the outfit. Even a change of jewelry or a new scarf can give you a fresh look.

What Does Your Wardrobe Say About You?

If you have any questions about your own sense of style, just look at the clothes in your closet—the fabrics, the colors, the cuts, the combinations. What you wear most often is indicative of your personal style, whether you're conscious of it or not.

Excluding your work wardrobe, examine what you have in your closets. If most of the garments before you are informal—jeans and flannel shirts, for example—your personal style reflects your desire for a casual life. Lots of sexy black dresses and sleek slacks with silk tops point to a penchant for nights on the town.

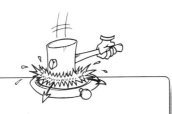

Time Stopper

Here's an easy way to give new life to your wardrobe. Break up your suits. Rather than wearing the same blouse with a suit every time you put it on, pair the jacket with a dress instead of its matching skirt. On another day, top the skirt with a contrasting sweater set. Nothing dates you more than wearing an outfit the exact same way every time.

Look at your sweaters: Do you have more cable knits and loose-fitting crewnecks, or is there a predominance of matching sweater sets and jeweled shrugs? One look is neither right nor wrong. It merely indicates your personal style.

Does Your Style Date You?

Soon we'll start you out on a Blitz of your entire wardrobe. For now, we only want you to be aware of the clothing that you've chosen and why you like it. We haven't yet asked you to consider if your choices make you feel and look young or old, or if they are current or dated.

It takes the scrutiny of a Blitz to answer those questions.

With a Blitz, you are confronted with probing questions. You will have to decide which, if any, of your choices make you look like you're stuck in time. This isn't a simple case of like or dislike, but a matter of how young your wardrobe makes you look and feel right now.

Why Did I Buy That?

Look in the farthest, darkest corner of your closet. If you're anything like us, you'll find the fashion mistakes you've made over the years. This might be something you bought on sale because the clerk said it made you look so young. It could be a fantastic dress that you had planned to wear after you lost 20 pounds. It could even be a hip outfit in the J. Crew catalog that you couldn't wait to send for.

You might also have three black blazers, none of which is exactly right, which means you'll probably be buying a fourth before the year is over.

Starting to sound familiar? This is your wake-up call to start weeding through your wardrobe to determine whatever doesn't flatter you, things that are too sexy, too small, too trendy, or simply that no longer fit your lifestyle or your body.

What Are You Hanging On To?

Over the years, on countless shopping trips, you've made selections, most of which pleased you at the time. As we've mentioned, many of them are still hanging in your closet or stuffed into your chest of drawers, unworn.

Look carefully at them now. Do you really want them? Probably not. As soon as you acknowledge that the only thing they do is take up space, you'll be able to get rid of them. You may be surprised by the realization that you have been hanging on to things you wore when you were younger because they once made you feel terrific.

Don't hold on to your youth that has passed. It only makes you feel old. Create a new youth for the new you.

By the end of this chapter, you just might be able to reach into any corner of your closet and find something to wear that will suit you perfectly, combining comfort, fit, and a fresh new look.

It won't be cluttered with clothing and accessories you never use.

The next time you go on a shopping spree, you will be ready to look at yourself with fresh eyes and choose clothing befitting the vibrant, youthful person you are becoming.

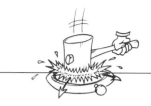

Time Stopper

If you're at all puzzled about what to keep and what to throw away, call on a friend whose taste in clothing you admire and whose opinions you trust. Be ready to be laughed at. Things you thought were amazing when you bought them may range from dated to ridiculous. Your friend will let you know. Don't be insulted; just take the advice and throw the stuff out. Then thank your brave friend.

You're Not Alone

Lest you start feeling guilty about hanging on to clothes long past their prime, and even those that never had one, here are our confessions.

Sallie had an emerald-green silk shantung cocktail dress, worn once before she moved to New York in the early 1970s. She never had occasion to wear it again, yet every time she saw it, she recalled how wonderful she had felt when she wore it. Besides, it was the size she wanted to be, so every once in a while she hauled it out for a size check. Finally, while cleaning out her closets before a paint job, she tossed it into the Goodwill pile. It had gone in and out of style so many times that it needed a rest. "I was amazed at how good it felt to clear it out of my life. I'd moved so far beyond it I never realized that I didn't need it anymore."

Hattie has a long, elegant lace nightgown that she bought about five years ago for her fantasy trousseau. Mind you, she wasn't even in a relationship at the time. "I try on clothes and even buy them to wardrobe my dreams. That way, when they come true—and they often do—I always have something beautiful to wear." The lace nightie is still hanging in her closet, ready to be worn.

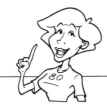

Voice of Experience

"The beauty of a woman is not in the clothes she wears, the figure that she carries, or the way she combs her hair. The beauty of a woman must be seen in her eyes, because that is the doorway to her heart, the place where love resides."

—Audrey Hepburn, *Speaking on Beauty*

Defining an Ageless Look

An ageless look is in style when you're 30 … and when you're 60. It has no time attached to it. You'll never be able to peg a date on it, nor will it tell your age.

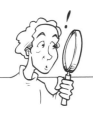

Age Alert

The fashion magazines aren't the only place to get pointers on what's new and stylish. Watch TV and movies … and check out celebrities at work and at play. Chic doesn't have to be costly. Remember when Sharon Stone showed up at the Academy Awards wearing a crisp white T-shirt with a simple long skirt? She made headlines!

Consider some of the perennial beauties—Jacqueline Kennedy Onassis, Audrey Hepburn, Princess Diana, Sophia Loren, Lena Horne. Each in her own personal style achieved an ageless look that surpasses time.

Let's not forget the men. While gray hair and character lines are more acceptable for men, they can still be defined by an ageless look. Consider Cary Grant, Paul Newman, Sean Connery, Larry King and his suspenders, and Regis Philbin, who becomes more debonair each year.

What sets these public figures apart is their strong connection with their bodies and their beings. They wear their clothing, not the other way around. They exude a confidence that transcends time.

Take Audrey Hepburn, for example. She chose clothing with simple, sleek lines with few extraneous details. She stayed with solids over patterns and opted for a timeless, classic look. This became her trademark.

Such simplicity of style is ageless. We can learn from her example.

An Ageless Look of Your Own

Following the lead of these stylish celebrities, you can create an ageless look that keeps you timeless and young. This personal style incorporates the qualities you value and have cultivated your entire life. It matches who you are, deep down. It's as individual as a fingerprint.

Unity of style and spirit comes only when you develop a powerful sense of who you are as a human being. Then you will be able to dress that human being—who happens to be you—in a manner that honors the dignity and beauty of who you have become. True youth is borne by the spirit. It comes from within, rather than a certain article of clothing or a fashionable accessory.

From this new perspective filled with self-respect, look through your wardrobe and eliminate everything that is not in keeping with the special person you've become.

Don't overlook clothing that may look beautiful but feels awful. Clothing that constricts your body and inhibits movement makes you feel awkward and old. Select clothes that move freely with the body so that you'll feel youthful and graceful.

Time to Blitz ... Again

You'll have to muster up a lot of courage to tackle this task. No other area of our lives is more charged than our appearance. We fall on insults and rise on compliments. Now we're asking you to become brutally critical of the choices you've made to adorn your body.

You love many of these choices. In fact, you've become attached to them. We bet you that there's some item of clothing—a sweater, a piece of jewelry, a special outfit—that brings up a wellspring of memories every time you see it. You may even be able to recite every time you wore it, recounting in minute detail when and where you bought it ... or the lover who gave it to you.

Such memories, though cherished, tie us to our past. To be truly young and in the moment requires that we become unfettered. We admit that we're handing you a tough assignment, but we assert that only by bravely blitzing can we move forward in our lives.

Time to break out the heavy-duty trash bags and sturdy boxes. A reminder: The bags are for garbage, and the boxes go to the homeless shelter or charity of your choice.

Put on your favorite CD and get to work.

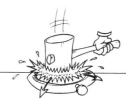

Time Stopper

Even if something was very expensive, if it doesn't make you feel like a million bucks every time you put it on, get rid of it.

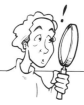

Age Alert

Remember: Blitzing is an ongoing process. What is a possible keeper today might be a throwaway tomorrow.

Just as you did when you blitzed your cosmetics, you'll be deciding what to toss, what to give away, and what to keep. This won't be easy. Blitzing something as personal as the clothes on your back can tap into deep feelings of loss and deprivation. That's probably why we hold on to so much stuff.

To Toss or Not To Toss?

To simplify this Blitz, think of what's before you in three categories: Throwaways; Giveaways, and Keepers. Notice: We have not suggested an "I'll Think It Over" heading. We want you to be bold and decisive.

➤ **Throwaways.** These are immediately obvious … or should be. Anything that's too worn, stained, and otherwise unwearable goes into the garbage. If you can't trust yourself to toss that soft tee shirt that's so worn you can read through it but feels so good when you sleep in it, imagine your lover—or your employer—surprising you when you're wearing it. Doesn't that help with your decision?

➤ **Giveaways.** If it's too good to toss but no longer enhances your wardrobe or your life, give it away. It may not suit you anymore, but it could be perfect for someone else. Knowing you've moved past a certain stage helps you pass these once-prized items on to someone who can appreciate them now.

➤ **Keepers.** Heading this list are items that absolutely delight you. You're happy that you bought them, and you're happy every time you wear them. There's no hesitation here. Pragmatically speaking, however, you may want to include as possible keepers skirts you can shorten, items you can update with color and youthful accessories, and anything you can't bear to part with right now.

All to the Mall

Once you've blitzed, you'll probably have lots of room in your closets. Now it's time for a shopping spree. Treat yourself to something new. Don't be afraid to experiment, being careful that you don't repeat your past mistakes, otherwise you'll end up with a closet filled with new throwaways and giveaways you'll never wear.

The key is to feel good about how you look.

Here are some ways to keep your wardrobe—and you—young and fresh:

➤ "Age-appropriate" doesn't have to mean stodgy and stiff. Generally speaking, don't dress like a teenager unless you are one.

➤ Exception to this rule: If a garment designed for a teen looks and feels great on you, wear it anyway.

➤ Pay attention to the proportion of your garments and accessories. Scale them toyour size. A petite woman will be dwarfed by a huge shawl; a large woman looks silly with a tiny handbag.

➤ Pick colors that complement your skin tone. Rule of thumb: When considering whether or not to buy something, hold it next to your face in front of a well-lit mirror. If it doesn't make your skin glow, the color's not for you, even though you really like it.

➤ Wear clothes that are comfortable but never shabby. Pay attention to your appearance, even when you're hanging out.

➤ Ask a sales clerk whose style you admire to pick out an outfit for you. Try it on before deciding whether it's for you. Often this person's suggestions turn out great and open you to a new way of dressing.

➤ Buy only clothes that fit you at the moment you try them on or require only simple alteration. Anything more than shortening a hem or moving a button is too much. Otherwise, they'll only haunt you as they hang in your closet unworn, waiting to be altered or for you to lose weight. Don't put that kind of pressure on yourself.

➤ Avoid the hottest trends; they'll only date you. This year's newest color or cut will be "last year's look" in a matter of months.

The Least You Need to Know

➤ Fashions often change with the whims of designers.

➤ Style travels elegantly through time.

➤ An ageless look is connected to a person's truest self.

➤ Your personal style defines who you are and how you feel.

➤ Blitzing your wardrobe provides constant renewal.

➤ Updating your look keeps you looking and feeling young.

Part 3

Looking and Feeling Young with E.A.S.E.

You can liken the road to youth to a four-lane expressway, each with its own E.A.S.E. pass. To help you on your way, we've broken the essential steps to growing younger into four categories:

E = EXERCISE   A = ATTITUDE   S = SKINCARE   E = EATING

The catch is there's no passing lane. You've got to approach all four essentials with equal dedication. One element is not more important than the others.

Daily focus on each category guarantees a radical shift in your aging process. This part—E.A.S.E.—provides the road map for your adventure in growing younger.

E is for EXERCISE. In addition to providing you with a matrix for a body of exercises that will help you feel fit and fabulous, we give you a program we call BEDCERCISE™. This program consists of easy-to-do, yet highly effective, stretches you can do in the relaxed atmosphere of your bedroom.

A is for ATTITUDE. Expanding on the Self-Image/Self-Esteem Connection introduced in Chapter 9, you'll get a boost in the attitude department, learning even more ways to change your aging as you change the way you think.

S is for SKINCARE. The importance of skincare, although often overlooked or at least downplayed, is vital to your age-reversing process. We take it far beyond how to wash your face and into the realm of regeneration. We even give you an exercise regime specifically for your face called Lift Your Face™.

E is for EATING. No one can deny that eating is one of the most important aspects of staying young. Adopting a new approach to food will change your eating habits for life. We'll introduce several great ideas in this part before devoting Part 4 in its entirety to "Putting Youth on Your Plate."

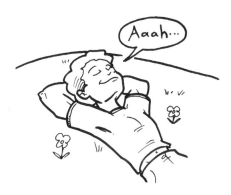

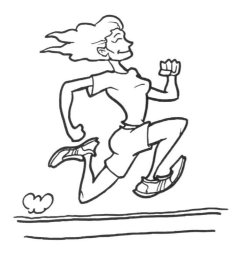

Chapter 11

E = EXERCISE to Feel Fit and Fabulous

In This Chapter

➤ Learning the secret of a child's energy

➤ Revealing how you keep fit ... or do you?

➤ Making fitness fun

➤ Measuring resting and target heart rates

➤ Discovering water aerobics and other alternatives to the gym

The first E of your E.A.S.E. program stands for Exercise.

Nowhere is the "use it or lose it" axiom more true than when it is applied to exercise. Exercising won't make you too tired to exercise, but lack of enough exercise will. What a vicious cycle.

If you don't like formal training or going to the gym, there are alternatives. There's dancing, swimming, long walks ... all sorts of activities that you can enjoy. Just make sure you do several forms of concentrated exercise *every single day*.

Frequency and variety are necessary to train your body to regenerate and provide you with youthful energy.

Where Do Children Get All That Energy?

Watch children. They seem inexhaustible. The reason is they keep moving. They aren't plagued by constant self-recriminations, either. You won't hear nine-year-olds complaining that they've got to quit eating so many carbs or sign up for a step aerobics class to fit into a new dress. They also aren't obsessed with their cholesterol levels, resting pulses, or whether they'll be admired for being a jock.

Don't Worry, Be Active

Simply put, kids don't worry. We do. They just want to have fun. And moving—a.k.a. exercising—is a favorite way of having a good time.

On the other hand, we adults often excuse our inactivity by saying, "I'm too tired to exercise." Fears of injury and illness also stifle our impulses to move and have fun. We replace exuberance with worry and become sedentary in the process. Not a good tradeoff.

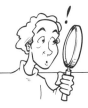

Age Alert

If walking is the only thing you do for fitness, you are not getting enough exercise to be young and healthy.

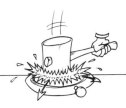

Time Stopper

Don't hold back from exercising for fear of injury or pain. Done properly, exercise doesn't create problems, it solves them. Be sure that you warm up adequately, and never force a movement.

The Freedom of Flexibility

Another major difference between children's bodies and adults' is that children move with abandon. They bend and unbend effortlessly, fall without serious injury, and romp with joy. Flexibility is never an issue.

By the time we reach our 20s (about the same time we start our careers), we find ourselves bound to a desk or on our feet at work all day. This gives us little time for active play. We notice that our muscles are tighter and our joints stiffer. That's when people start to move less. As a result, they become tighter and even less flexible. This in turn creates pain, and pain discourages movement.

This is why too many older adults—and also some who aren't so old—hesitate to do anything that requires more than minimal movement. They're constantly holding back in hopes of preventing injury and pain. Unfortunately, this too results in an unfit body that will age before its time.

S-t-r-e-t-c-h It Out

Stretching exercises break this destructive loop by releasing tension in the muscles and tendons around the joints. This increases the range of motion throughout your body, making you more sure-footed and agile.

When you've loosened up, you'll be less susceptible to injury and more able to romp like a child again.

Keeping Up with Keeping Fit

Look back at the Exercise Profile you developed in Chapter 5, "A Body of Exercise." You wrote down how much physical activity—formal and informal—you do every day. You also took a look at your body's response to this exercise and ranked your level of fitness from 1 to 10.

Am I as Fit as I Want to Be?

Now it's time to take a closer look at what you do to keep fit and to develop the most effective exercise program for your body and your age. You might want to write down your answers, or at least look at what you recorded in the BodyChecks you completed in Part 1, "Here's Looking at You." Here are some questions to ask yourself:

➤ When I exercise, do I keep the three essential keys—aerobics, flexibility, and strength—in mind? Which do I concentrate on and which do I overlook?

➤ What can I do to adjust my current exercise program so that it includes a balance of all three components?

➤ Does my exercise program leave me feeling exhausted or invigorated? In what ways?

➤ Do I allow my body adequate time to rest and recycle between exercise sessions?

➤ Does my current exercise program keep me at the level of fitness I want to be? If I am not at that level, is it sufficient to take me there?

➤ Besides my formal program, what activities do I do to keep fit?

➤ What are my fitness plans for the future?

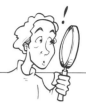

Age Alert

Before beginning any exercise program, get a physical checkup. This is absolutely essential, especially if you haven't had an exam during the past year and you aren't particularly physical in your day-to-day life. Other guidelines: Get a checkup if you're over 30; overweight; or have a history of high blood pressure, diabetes, or heart trouble. Don't just dive into vigorous activity. A thorough exam can help you avoid orthopedic injuries, cardiovascular complications, and other assorted exercise-related aches and pains.

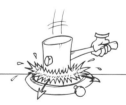

Time Stopper

When watching TV, get in the habit of doing some exercise during commercial breaks. Run in place instead of to the fridge, or just get up and stretch.

More Measures of Fitness

Fitness cannot be measured by appearances alone.

How much you weigh, the size of your waistline, how energetic and alert you are, and how well you sleep at night are not the ways to measure your fitness level—they're the rewards.

Resting Heart Rate

One excellent gauge of physical capacity is your resting heart rate. Between 65 and 80 beats per minute is excellent at any age.

Here's how to measure it: Take your pulse as soon as you wake up in the morning, before you get out of bed. Count the number of beats for 10 seconds, and then multiply that by six. This gives you your pulse in beats per minute. Do this for two mornings, and then calculate the average of the two. This figure is your resting heart rate.

Take your resting heart rate every three to four months to keep tabs on where you are.

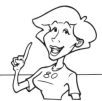

Voice of Experience

Sticking to it is probably the most difficult part of any exercise program. In case you haven't heard, your neighborhood health club is probably *counting* on you to drop out. Most spas are oversold by 300 percent or more because so many members simply quit coming before their memberships expire.

Your Target Heart Rate

When beginning an exercise program, it's helpful to have a target heart rate to measure your aerobic capacity. Here's the formula:

1. Take your resting pulse. Subtract that number from 220 beats per minute. This is your *maximum attainable heart rate*.

2. Subtract your age from 220 beats per minute. That's called your *heart rate reserve*.

3. Subtract your resting pulse from that figure.

4. If you are a beginning exerciser, multiply the resulting number by 60 percent. If you're a regular exerciser, multiply by 75 percent. If you're a competitive athlete (that means an Olympian or pro basketball player, not someone who works up a sweat once a week playing handball), multiply by 80 percent. This final figure is your *target heart rate.*

For maximum aerobic benefit, maintain your target heart rate for 20 minutes at least three times a week.

What's the Condition of Your Conditioning Program?

The conditioning component of your exercise program deals with flexibility, muscle strength, and endurance. Since each is important, you need a balanced exercise package for complete conditioning.

Include aerobic exercise for the cardiovascular endurance necessary to resist general fatigue, strength training for increased muscle power and endurance, and stretching to make sure you can use your strength and endurance without injury.

Having Fun Yet?

Exercise is one of those things people often do for the result, not for the fun of it. That's why so many join health clubs, only to quit going after a month or two. It's also why they buy closets full of equipment, only to let it gather dust.

Once a good idea has worn off, or the desired result is reached, it's easy to put exercise on the back burner or even stop.

Looking Forward to Exercise

Choose activities that are both enjoyable and productive so that you'll look forward to doing them. Otherwise, you probably won't continue for long, or worse, you *will* continue, but at the expense of your pleasure.

The most effective fitness plan resonates with who you are. Don't force yourself to fit into someone else's program. It's not good exercise to get bent out of shape!

The ideal routine allows you to adjust the pace to your individual ability. You should be able to step up the pace or ease off if you need to.

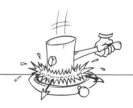

Time Stopper

Weight training is not just the best way to develop muscle mass and strength. It has been proven to retard bone loss and increase bone density, preventing osteoporosis.

Resisting Those Infomercial Miracles

Have you ever been dazzled by the promises of some super-fit exercise guru or beautiful model on one of those late-night infomercials? They can certainly be convincing—especially when you're only half awake. And they make it so easy with their money-back guarantees and sincere testimonials.

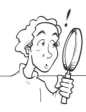

Age Alert

When joining a gym or exercise program, make sure that it takes the abilities of its participants into consideration. You will be likely to drop out if a class is so slow or easy that it's boring, or so fast that you have trouble keeping up. Also, you may injure yourself if the exercise is too difficult.

It's easy to get hooked. Even savvy, health-conscious people who *know* there are no shortcuts to fitness buy the line. For example, one very fit woman in her 60s is a chronic insomniac and watches TV well into the night when the channels are flooded with pitches for miracle-producing exercise equipment. She was captivated by a complete gym gizmo that promised total fitness in only six minutes a day, payable in 36 easy payments. She took the bait. When the apparatus arrived, it was huge. And it was heavy. Its very presence in the corner of her bedroom nagged at her. "I knew I would have to force myself to use it and couldn't wait to get it out of my house," she confesses.

"It would have taken me more than six minutes a day just to set the thing up," she laughs. "Thank goodness I had the presence of mind to save the packaging. It cost me a bundle just to send it back! I've learned my lesson about buying things in the middle of the night. I'm going to stick with swimming and ballroom dancing, things I love to do."

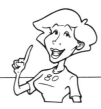

Voice of Experience

Forget the maxim "No pain, no gain."

Experts—from sports physicians to phys. ed. teachers—say emphatically that the most important principle of safe training is if something you're doing hurts, stop doing it. Pain is one of the body's ways of signaling to you that it is being injured.

Fitness Trends

You can't turn on the television or pick up a magazine without seeing some new fitness craze. Most come and go, but others have become part of the smorgasbord of exercise styles available to you.

New routines, such as step aerobics and Tae-Bo, have jumped their way onto the schedules of fitness centers around the world. Others, like yoga and belly dancing, have been with us for centuries.

Try Something New

Check the schedules at your gym or community center, and look into local adult education programs, such as the Seminar Center, Learning Annex, and Learning Studio. You just may find introductory classes so you can sample several different styles—Pilates, spinning, swing dancing—until you find one that appeals to you.

Try something completely new. Experimentation keeps you youthful.

If Classes Aren't for You

Even if being super fit isn't your goal, you'll never look and feel young without exercise. How can an ordinary person who simply wants to drop a few pounds and feel fit be expected to stick to an exercise plan?

Not everyone is inspired to work up a sweat in a brightly mirrored room pulsing with loud music. Some may even be intimidated when surrounded by fit bodies clad in Spandex. One solution would be to hire a personal trainer sensitive to your needs and abilities who will work one-on-one with you, either at the gym or at your home.

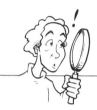

Age Alert

An exercise class needs more than a great body at the front of the room and a tape of dance music. Check out the teacher's training and experience. Talk to people who have taken classes with that instructor.

Then look at the facility, especially the floor. It should be firm yet resilient, made of wood with an airspace or spring cushion underneath, with mats for floor work.

Also look at ventilation, elbow room, and routine warm-ups and cool-downs.

Do you feel relaxed and energized after class?

Bringing the Gym to You

Your trainer can also help you stay on an exercise schedule and regulate your progress. A competent professional will design a program that suits *all* of your needs and motivates you to continue. This partnership also makes exercise much more enjoyable.

Another idea is to enroll a friend—or friends—in your exercise program. Make it a social event. Consider exploring area parks by foot or bicycle. Break your routine by changing your route every few days.

Everybody into the Pool!

An outstanding alternative to traditional exercise, water exercise, is growing in popularity among people of all ages and fitness levels. It's done in the shallow end of the pool, in waist- or chest-deep water, so you don't have to be a swimmer to reap the rewards of this exercise, which is rooted in physical therapy and sports medicine.

You weigh 90 percent less in water than you do on dry land. As a consequence, people who find it difficult to jog or jump or perform other weight-bearing exercises are able to work out with ease when buoyed by water.

Whether you call it aquatic exercise, aquarobics, water jogging, or any other name, water exercise is the perfect low-impact aerobic activity, safe enough for arthritis sufferers.

Check your local YMCA or community center for pool exercise programs.

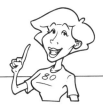

Voice of Experience

Hattie discovered water exercises in her 60s. "I'd been taking and teaching exercise and dance classes for more than 45 years. I wanted to try something new, so when I saw that my health club was offering water exercise classes, I enrolled in a heartbeat. I've always loved the water, so I figured this might be fun. I love it. Now I go four to five times a week. There's nothing like seeing myself in a bathing suit to keep me on my toes."

Take a Hike

Probably the most natural and least-expensive form of exercise possible, walking builds stamina and helps to relieve tension, enhances muscle tone, and improves cardiovascular fitness. Almost anyone—even the very obese—can do it with relative ease.

Maximize the benefits—and raise the comfort level—of your walking workout by wearing a good pair of walking or running shoes that fit without rubbing and provide sufficient arch support. Before striking out, take a few minutes to stretch your hamstrings and Achilles tendons, then warm up by walking slowly for the first two to three minutes of your walk.

Practice maintaining good posture, keeping your head up, shoulders back, and arms swinging freely at your sides. Step down on the back of your heels and roll forward onto your toes. Breathe deeply and exhale fully as you walk. Slow your pace for the last three to five minutes to cool down.

There's only one catch: Walking is not enough to provide a full workout, so make sure you round it out with strength training and stretches.

A Bit About Biking

Cycling can do wonders for body and soul. It gets you out in the fresh air and really gets your heart and lungs working, leaving you feeling fully energized.

Before you start out, get a bicycling helmet in a bright color—so motorists can see you. In some areas, cycling helmets are required by law. Make sure your helmet is constructed of hard plastic or polycarbonate with a stiff polystyrene lining and has a securely attached nylon strap and fastener. Look for a label stating that the American Standards Institute or the Snell Memorial Foundation certifies the headgear as safe. Then make sure you use it.

Age Alert

For you indoor bikers: For safety's sake, make certain that the stationary bike standing in the corner of your bedroom—under all those clothes—is as sturdy as a road racer. The view may not be as verdant as a leafy bike path, but the workout *is* every bit as effective.

You can't just ride *any* bike. It has to be right for your size. You should be able to sit on the seat and put one foot on the ground without leaning the bike to one side or the other.

The bike shop can adjust the seat and handlebars for a proper fit. The seat should be placed so that when one leg is extended and bent slightly, the ball of your foot contacts the pedal at the lowest point of its revolution. Handlebars should be no lower than the seat.

Winter Workouts

Cold-weather exercise seems to burn more fat than that sweaty game of volleyball on the beach. Studies at the School of Physical and Health Education at the University of Toronto show that one advantage of exercising in the cold is the mobilization of fat. More fat is burned during cold-weather workouts than in the more temperate seasons—in part, because of the need to generate body heat.

Cross-country skiing tops the list of effective wintertime exercises. It works the upper and lower body simultaneously, building strength in the arms and legs and providing the heart and lungs with an outstanding workout. Snowshoeing is right behind cross-country skiing in its aerobic intensity.

If the cold is unbearable, consider using a Nordic Track, which simulates the movements of cross-country skiing without the goosebumps.

The Least You Need to Know

➤ Children's energy comes naturally; adults have to work for it.

➤ If your fitness plan doesn't fit you, find one that does.

➤ Your resting and target heart rate are measures of your level of aerobic fitness.

➤ Choosing a program that's fun will keep you coming back for more.

➤ Exercising in a pool is one of the safest, most enjoyable ways to keep fit.

➤ There's a smorgasbord of fitness options out there—some old (yoga), some new (Tae-Bo). Give them a try.

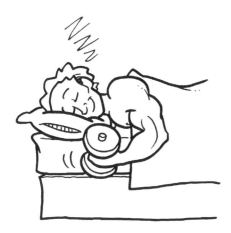

Chapter 12

BEDCERCISE™— the Lazy Way to Lifelong Flexibility

In This Chapter

➤ The lazy way to fitness

➤ BEDCERCISES™ are for everyone

➤ Wake up and move

➤ Bedtime stretches to help you sleep

➤ No strain, much gain

Hattie has been teaching dance and exercise for more than 45 years and is in fabulous shape. So, one might assume that she loves to exercise. "No way," she protests. "I find ways to be fit without forcing myself to exercise."

Hattie describes how—just like in Marlene Dietrich's song, "I'm the Laziest Gal in Town" —she went from her two favorite bed exercises, phoning for Chinese food and dusting for crumbs, to a series of highly effective, safe, and fun exercises to be done in bed.

Sallie, who just might be the second laziest gal in town, had been exercising in bed for years, stretching and getting ready for another sedentary day at her desk.

We both start our mornings with energizing exercises that wake up our joints and muscles and then end each day with stress-releasing stretches in bed. Ironically, we had begun doing them independently of the other and only discovered it when talking how we'd been soothing our aching joints.

Bed Exercises— Are You Kidding?

Why not? We spend almost a third of our lives in bed. It's where we begin and end each day.

BEDCERCISES are as stress-free as exercise can get.

You don't need to get up and go anywhere. You need no special apparatus, clothing (whatever you sleep in is fine), or even skill. Presumably, there are no distractions … and surely there is no competition, no noise, and no instructor telling you what to do next. You have the luxury of exercising in your most private, secure environment, in your own time, at your own speed.

No equipment is involved, so you can do these exercises no matter where you are. Man or woman, old or young, fit or not-so-fit, these exercises are suited for anyone.

Easy Does It

BEDCERCISES are totally safe, because they place no stress or pressure on the musculoskeletal system. They also reduce pain in the joints and muscles, even if caused by *arthritis*, and help prevent and heal injuries.

These simple movements encourage you to become attuned to your physical, emotional, and spiritual being, achieving balance and unity.

While not a *substitute* for either aerobic exercise, which builds heart-lung function, or weight-bearing activity, for bone density, BEDCERCISES add the benefit of lifelong flexibility. Ironically, both aerobic and weight-bearing exercise diminish flexibility. BEDCERCISES provide a necessary antidote.

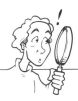

Age Alert

Don't get hurt. Everyone who engages in strong physical activity, either at work or play, needs to keep his or her joints supple. Add exercises for flexibility to your program so that you don't set yourself up for injury. This is especially true if you concentrate on strength training and high-impact aerobics.

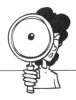

WatchWord

BEDCERCISES are highly effective, stress-free exercises that are done in bed. When done in the morning before arising and again at bedtime, they increase flexibility of the joints and muscles.

The best part is that this easy, pleasant ritual helps retard and reverse the aging process and keeps you flexible forever.

Besides, it's fun.

First Thing in the Morning

Doing your BEDCERCISES each morning provides an invigorating transition from sleep to wakefulness. They prepare the body for the rigors of the day ahead and lubricate the joints with *synovial fluid* so that you don't sound like popcorn when you get out of bed.

Last Thing at Night

Done at bedtime, these very same exercises relieve the tension and stress accumulated during the course of the day. They will become an easy, pleasant ritual to end the day. Another plus: They guarantee a restful night's sleep.

BEDCERCISE contradicts the commonly held belief that exercise should not be done before going to sleep. These stress-reducing movements, combined with relaxing, sleep-inducing breath work, will send you off to dreamland.

Make It Your Own

You can customize this program to your individual needs. If you have limited mobility, trauma after injury, long- and short-term confinements to bed, or are recuperating after illness or surgery, do as much or as little as feels comfortable.

As you grow healthier and more flexible, you may find that you will be able to do these exercises more fully.

BEDCERCISES for Flexibility

These gentle movements pack a wallop. Here are five bed exercises that are all you need to maintain young and flexible joints.

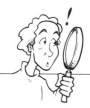

Age Alert

If you lift weights for strength without balancing your program with equally intense flexibility work, you run the risk of becoming a muscle-bound hulk. You may look cut and buff, but you'll be stiff as a robot.

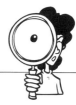

WatchWord

Arthritis—the stiffening and inflammation of joints—is the second-largest health problem among older people, second only to hearing loss. By age 30 (yes, that young), 35 percent of the population is plagued by osteo-arthritis. Exercising in bed can minimize both pain and damage from this potentially debilitating malady.

Synovial fluid is the body's "motor oil" that keeps our joints moving smoothly and without friction. Produced by the synovium membrane that surrounds our joints or tendons, it not only lubricates surrounding surfaces but also nourishes these tissues.

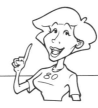

Voice of Experience

"You are as young as your joints," says Hattie, explaining how exercising in bed reverses and retards the stiffness often associated with aging. "I started exercising in bed to relieve the awful pains I was feeling in my shoulders and lower back from my body therapy work. It got me out of bed in the morning, ready to take on another day of arduous physical activity. When I skipped my BEDCERCISES, I felt stiff and achy all day."

The Crossover Stretch

Purpose: To release tension in the lower back and hip sockets; to prevent injury by increasing flexibility of the spine.

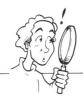

Age Alert

Stretch as far as you are able without forcing. In time, you may find that you can extend these moves to the max.

Starting position: Flat on your back, hands at your sides.

Step 1: Bend right knee to chest. With left hand, gently pull your bent leg across your body to the right.

Step 2: Hold this position for a slow count of five, making sure that you breathe deeply.

Step 3: Straighten leg and return to starting position.

Step 4: Repeat with left leg.

Repetitions: 3

The crossover stretch.

(Photo by Bill Miller)

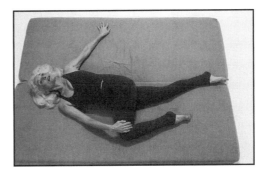

The Hip Releaser

Purpose: To release tension in the hip sockets and lower back; to stretch the inner thighs.

Starting position: Lie flat on your back, arms outstretched at shoulder level.

> **Step 1:** Bend knees, keeping legs together and feet flat on the bed.
>
> **Step 2:** Let legs fall apart as far as you can into an open diamond shape, putting your feet together, sole to sole. Hold for a count of five.
>
> **Step 3:** Pull legs back together, keeping knees bent.
>
> **Step 4:** Slowly roll legs from side to side, getting as close to the bed as possible with each roll.
>
> **Step 5:** Return to starting position.

Repetitions: 5

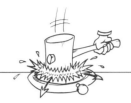

Time Stopper

The slow twisting action of this crossover stretch releases tension from the intricate network of muscles and supportive ligaments surrounding the spine. By targeting the connective tissue of the lumbar vertebrae of the lower back, this exercise prevents injuries and alleviates stiffness and chronic pain.

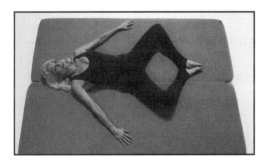

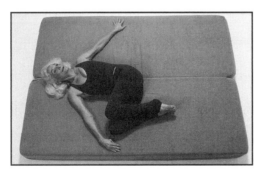

The hip releaser.

(Photo by Bill Miller)

123

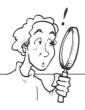

Age Alert

The hips bear the brunt of many of the pressures our body faces throughout our lives. High-impact activities, such as active sports and jogging, place undue wear and tear on these ball-and-socket joints. Worn-down heels, as well as high heels, that throw the body off-balance compound the problem. Don't overlook the need for tension-releasing exercises and massage to take the pressure off these overstressed joints.

The Leg Pull-Up

Purpose: To release tension in the lower back; to keep knee joints and hip sockets flexible; to enhance range of motion and stretch hamstrings.

Starting position: Flat on your back, hands at your sides.

Step 1: Keeping legs together, bend knees and clasp your hands behind your thighs. Pull knees up as close to your chest as you can.

Step 2: Still supporting your thighs with your clasped hands, straighten legs. Hold for a count of five.

Step 3: Point, then flex toes 10 times. Breathe deeply and fully as you hold this position.

Step 4: Bend legs and slowly return to starting position.

Repetitions: 5

The leg pull-up.

(Photo by Bill Miller)

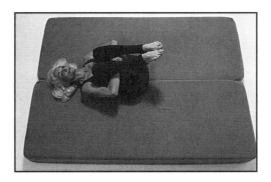

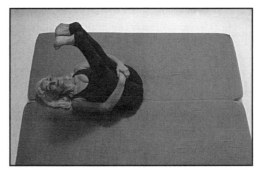

The Prone Stretch

Purpose: To stretch the neck, chest, arms, and torso; to strengthen the buttocks.

Starting position: Stretch out face-down on the bed, arms at your sides.

Step 1: Move hands to shoulder level, bending elbows and pressing palms flat into the bed.

Step 2: Straighten arms as in a pushup, lifting your head and raising your shoulders from the mattress. Your back will arch. Tighten your buttocks.

Step 3: Point your toes. Keeping the tops of your feet flat on the bed, continue stretching your torso upward as far as possible. Look up toward the ceiling.

Step 4: Hold for a count of 10, then slowly lower your body until you are lying flat on the bed. Make sure that you don't hold your breath.

Step 5: Return to your starting position.

Repetitions: 5

Time Stopper

Remember: Never hold your breath. When the instructions say "hold for a count of 10," that means you should hold that *position,* not your *breath.* This applies to any form of exercise you do.

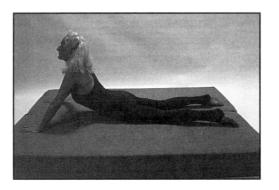

The prone stretch.

(Photo by Bill Miller)

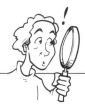

Age Alert

Poor posture can affect your lung capacity. When we sit and walk, we often let our chest cave in and our shoulders slouch forward. To counter this compression, stretches that lift the rib cage and open the chest are essential. That's what the prone and ultimate stretches accomplish. Do them daily.

The Ultimate Stretch

Purpose: To stretch the neck, chest, arms, and torso; to strengthen the buttocks.

Starting position: Seated, upright, with legs spread as far apart as comfortable.

Step 1: Place hands on bed in front of body. Slide hands and arms to the front as you lean forward as far as you can bend without forcing. Make certain that you breathe slowly and deeply.

Step 2: Clasp hands behind your back, and pull your shoulder blades together.

Step 3: Slowly return to upright sitting position. Continue to extend clasped hands to the back, extending arms as straight as possible.

Step 4: Release and return to starting position.

Repetitions: 3

The ultimate stretch.

(Photo by Bill Miller)

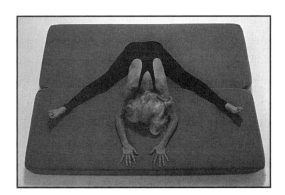

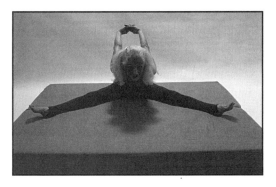

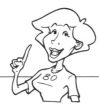

Voice of Experience

New York massage therapist Joel Benjamin, whose client list reads like a who's who in theater and dance, advises, "Whenever you feel a pull or tightness in a muscle while exercising, it's a good idea to stop and massage that spot before going on. Dancers are so intent on getting through a routine that they often forget to take time to take care of their muscles. A few minutes of massage while warming up can prevent long-term damage later on."

Most people never think in terms of doing exercises—other than the obvious—in bed. By including BEDCERCISE in your daily age-reversing program, you are introducing your body to a whole new way of being fit.

The Least You Need to Know

➤ Even lazy people can exercise in bed.

➤ Even the simplest exercises give you fitness benefits.

➤ When exercising, remember to breathe.

➤ Daily stretching prevents injury.

➤ BEDCERCISE is fun.

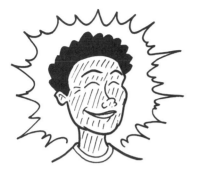

A = ATTITUDES That Keep You Young

> ## In This Chapter
>
> ➤ Beliefs about aging
>
> ➤ Your honest feelings about how you've aged
>
> ➤ Was being young really so great?
>
> ➤ Negative thinking sabotages youth
>
> ➤ Developing a positive view
>
> ➤ Affirmations for a new attitude

The A in E.A.S.E. stands for Attitude. Attitude underscores every aspect of reversing aging. Nothing else determines how you feel about yourself as powerfully as your belief system.

We were all born young, weren't we? So why have so many of us become old before our time? And why are we afraid of aging?

It Started in Childhood

We've been brainwashed since we were children to believe that old age is unappealing, undesirable, and physically unattractive. Hardly a day goes by that we're not subjected to some snide comment or ugly image about an older person.

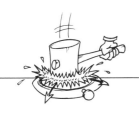

Time Stopper

Face your fears about growing old. That's the only way to overcome them and reverse your aging process. Fear is aging.

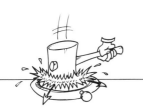

Time Stopper

True youth is vibrancy, energy, courage, joyfulness, and openness. Time does not destroy our innate ability to generate these qualities. A young spirit is ageless.

We are deluged with the appeal of youth, as if only the young have value. To be a young person is admirable; to be an old person is repugnant. This message is delivered over and over again at every turn.

What Does "Old" Mean, Anyway?

According to *Webster's New Universal Unabridged Dictionary*, the first definition of the word "old" is pretty benign: "1. Advanced far in years; having lived beyond the middle period, or toward the end of the ordinary term of living; aged …."

After that, things get defamatory: "2. Having been in use for a long time; shabby; trite; worn out; decayed by time."

How's that for inspiration?

Our language abounds with derogatory illusions: Old maid. Old goat. Old fogy. Old hat. Old crone. Old wife. Old codger.

Consequently, in our culture, it's a rare soul who relishes living past his or her "prime." You don't hear about too many kids who aspire to be a wise old man with a cane. And we don't view that image in a positive light, either. That's why we must create our entire lives as "prime" time.

Age Is a Numbers Game

In this context, when we talk about being young, we're referring to calendar age, not frame of mind.

In a perfect world, who wouldn't wish for the wit and wisdom of their years all wrapped up in a 25-year-old body? Since that's not about to happen, we're better off accepting that we can't stop time. Rather than getting all worked up about age and numbers, we need to do all in our power to have the best possible physical package in which to play.

Your body is capable of continuous renewal. You needn't be 25 to feel energetic and appealing.

What Was So Great About Being Young, Anyway?

Instead of looking back and regretting the loss of youth, we must treasure the gift of time.

Anyone who stays hung up on memories of a glorious youth isn't in touch with reality. When memories are only of the high points (happy birthdays, first dates, great new jobs, and vacations at the beach), truth becomes distorted. What about the slights from people we thought were friends, the missed opportunities, the terror of going to war, broken promises that wounded us to the quick?

These were all part of youth, too.

Why are we so reluctant to admit that youth was not all parties and play? And why do we focus only on the downside of being older? All this does is set us up to be discontented with who we have become.

"If I Had Known Then What I Know Now"

Let's not forget how unsettled and unsure we were.

An accomplished music teacher who raised her family without household help recalls, "When I think back at how nervous, impatient, disorganized, and even hysterical I was when my children were small, I wonder how we survived."

She continues, "I wish I'd had the patience, dignity, and wisdom I have now. These qualities came with experience, and that took time. No wonder I cherish the aging process. It's made me the woman I always wanted to be."

Reflect on how your own life has spun into the present. No doubt the 20/20 vision of hindsight will enable you to see improvements that could have come only through time.

Don't Blame Aging

Stop viewing the past through rose-colored glasses and the future through gray-tinted bifocals.

In truth, there is little difference between being young and being old. Life is magnificent, and monstrous, at various turns. But as we keep searching for the reasons for our discontent, we automatically place the blame on aging.

Learn to stop blaming age for everything that goes wrong. Both youth and maturity have their share of problems and pleasures. It's natural to hang on to the happier moments. We are experts at denial

Time Stopper

Learn to focus your thoughts on things that are pleasant and productive. When you use your 13 billion brain cells for subjects that are creative, interesting, and funny, you will begin to feel better instantly.

and blocking out pain. It's been said that if women remembered the pain of child-birth, everyone would be an only child.

In what ways do you distort your past by believing that all opportunities and joys are behind you?

Clearly, there is no benefit in believing that the present is colorless, the future is bleak, and only the past has value. Yet we continue to cling to this way of thinking.

Get Excited!

Psychologist Dr. John Kildahl advises, "If you think that nothing excites you, that your prospects look bleak, that you will never reach your goals, that nothing you do will make any difference, then you are setting yourself for failure and for aging long before your time. Fortunately, that kind of thinking can be reversed at any age, whether one is 40, 50, 60, 70, 80, or even 90!"

He continues, "You can make life miserable with what you think, or you can free yourself to make the most of life's experiences and add excitement to your life."

Warped by Time

Preoccupation with aging and the anticipated horrors it brings creates an unhealthy psychological condition. We call this distorted thinking *time neurosis*.

Even the point at which one becomes "old" is subjective. One person may not consider herself old until she's well past 60, while another hits the age wall at 40, or even younger.

WatchWord

When a person becomes overly anxious with the prospect of growing old and the seeming loss of all vestiges of youth, the result can be debilitating. We call this preoccupation **time neurosis.**

Look into your own thoughts and feelings about aging. Acknowledge not only what bothers you or what you fear, but also what makes you happy and proud of yourself.

Too often we lose track of our good feelings in the avalanche of complaints that beg for attention.

You may have a great body but need to buy your pants one size larger. What happens? Instead of appreciating the fact that you're in terrific shape, you focus on your increased clothing size. This way of thinking sabotages youth.

How often have you done this to yourself?

Are you still doing it?

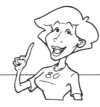

Voice of Experience

These warm words of wisdom from Dr. John Kildahl: "While you are relentless about ferreting out and eliminating your negative thoughts, please be very kind to yourself. Keep in mind whose side you are on. You are not the enemy. The enemy is your negative, depressing thoughts. You can be harsh with the unpleasant thoughts and stop them, but you don't have to extend that harshness to yourself. Be aware that you can always be your own best friend, as well as a kind, loving parent to yourself. Being kind to yourself will make differences in every aspect of your life."

Mind over Middle Age

Learn to use the power of your mind to create positive thoughts and images rather than wasting your energy by demeaning yourself.

Our nagging inner conversations are so pervasive that they can take control of our lives. Unless we take them in hand, we will become flooded with horrifying thoughts about ourselves and how we are aging.

This happens to everybody. For example, there was that night when you were all dressed up, ready to go out for a special occasion. Everything was perfect: sexy, low-cut gown, glamorous hairstyle, dazzling makeup. Then, under the bright lights over your bathroom sink, you noticed a few wrinkles and age spots framed by the deep V neckline of your gown. The inner voice delivers a whammy: "Good grief! You look so old. You're *way* too old to be wearing that dress. Who do you think you're trying to fool? Dress your age."

Suddenly, you felt deflated. It's like you've been punched in the gut. And an example for you men: You decide you're going to start playing tennis again. You were pretty good back in your 20s, but you haven't had time to play in years. You've gotten a new racquet and new tennis gear that makes you feel like Pete Sampras. You start the game, exhilarated by getting back on the court, when your attention is diverted. On the adjoining court are two young guys, agile and trim, running all over the court as they volley the ball.

Just like the woman in the gown, your inner voice pipes up: "You look ridiculous. It's about time you stop trying to be a young jock. You have no business trying to play tennis again. You're too out of shape."

Such self-inflicted cruelty will keep showing up unless you silence the voice and release its hold on you. It won't be quiet by itself. You must take action.

Speak Up!

The most effective antidote to this verbal self-abuse is a technique we call *attitude affirmations.* This process counters the negative thinking that robs us of our feelings of self-worth.

Attitude affirmations are your lifeline to youth.

An affirmation is simply a statement that shapes how we think. It transforms a negative thought by restating it in a positive context.

WatchWord

Attitude affirmations are powerful, positive statements that we say to ourselves to shatter our belief that we are no longer vital. They serve to silence the destructive inner voice that erodes our self-esteem as we age.

Because we are programmed to register only the bad stuff, we habitually disregard all the things we cherish about ourselves. Once again, our good qualities get short shrift.

It's important to admit that as we grow older, we repeatedly put ourselves down. If we truly want to look and feel younger, we must change this pattern by concentrating our energies on our attributes. Attitude affirmations accomplish this.

Curiously, facing the positive does not come naturally. It takes time to plant the idea of affirming the self. Continuous practice makes attitude affirmations an effective ally in your age-reversing program.

In developing our own age-reversing program, we devised the concept of attitude affirmations.

Attitude Affirmations—Lifeline to Youth

As you master this technique, you will add your own spin on the affirmation process. These are some affirmations we have found to be quite powerful:

➤ How I feel about aging will change with time. I can learn to appreciate and admire the very characteristics I now disdain.

➤ My body is a reflection of who I am. As I create myself to be a healthy, self-disciplined, and fine person, my look will reflect my being.

➤ It is not so much because I am aging that I look as I do ... it has more to do with how I have been treating myself.

➤ I can now treat myself exquisitely, no matter how I have treated myself and how others have treated me in the past.

➤ As I continue to take excellent care of myself, I will look and feel younger, more vital, and happier with each passing year.

➤ Society has handed me negative images of aging that have made me fear getting older. I refuse to buy into them.

➤ I will find my own personal style of experiencing aging so that I am excited at what the future holds.

➤ I can change my habitual negative habits of behavior and thought into positive, life-affirming ones.

And last but not least:

➤ I am not going to be a victim of my negativity, though I know it will persist in showing up.

Making Affirmations Work

Yes, negative thinking won't give up without a fight. Attitude affirmations provide you with the ammunition to beat it at its own game.

One way to fix your affirmations in your mind is to *write them down*. Use ones we suggested earlier, develop your own, or use a combination of both that works for you. Frame them in the present tense, using positive imagery to paint a clear and vivid picture of the result you want to achieve.

Then, whenever a negative thought enters your head, you'll have an arsenal of affirmations ready to use. Here's how the process works:

1. Acknowledge the negative thought. Don't attempt to repress it. Attempting to squelch it only makes it pop up later.

2. Counter it immediately with an appropriate attitude affirmation. Reach into your arsenal of affirmations, or make one up on the spot.

3. Repeat the affirmation until the negative thought disappears. You may have to do this several times for the positive statement to override the persistence of this negative thinking.

135

Caution: Negativity Ahead

Here are some do's and don'ts to keep in mind when trying to maintain a positive, youthful attitude:

➤ Don't expect your attitudes toward aging—and yourself—to change overnight. They've been around for eons and hold on for dear life.

➤ Don't allow backslides to stop you from your constant work; backslides are absolutely to be expected. Keep working in the face of them.

➤ Don't think you may be too old for really dramatic changes. Miracles happen at every stage of life.

➤ Consider that what you think about aging is based on your past and the history of our Western civilization. It may be entirely off the mark and ready for major revision, culturally and personally.

➤ Be prepared to give up old concepts, habits, and possessions. Holding on to things from the past keeps us mired in it.

➤ Expect to become depressed, disgusted, discouraged. Remember that discontent and disgust often provide a springboard for transformation to take place. We call this *creative self-disgust*.

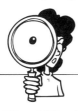

WatchWord

Creative self-disgust is a phrase we use to describe the use of self-criticism to inspire you to make changes that move your life forward.

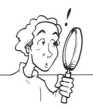

Age Alert

Every time you pick up something in yourself that you disapprove of, you react by blaming yourself for this flaw. Use creative self-disgust to motivate you to take corrective action.

Hattie's Special Attitude Boosters

Hattie calls her favorite attitude affirmations Hattietudes™. They give her an inspirational nudge to keep her spirits up and provide a potent, affirming quality. Like booster shots, they inject her with new energy that jolts her consciousness and stirs her to action.

She encourages her clients to tack their Hattietudes list on the wall beside their desks, on their refrigerator doors, or beside their bathroom mirrors, and to tuck them into their daily planners—places where they can get a lift from them throughout the day.

Here're some examples of her inspirational phrases:

- ➤ Impossible = I'm possible.
- ➤ Fighting Mother Nature is good exercise.
- ➤ Age is not the reason, it's the excuse.
- ➤ Remember the *you* in youth.
- ➤ The hands of time are yours. Take aging into your own hands.
- ➤ Life may get harder, but you get smarter.
- ➤ Convert envy into inspiration, and you'll never run out of fuel.
- ➤ Where there's a will there's a won't. Respect the negative.
- ➤ Bless every rejection. It takes hundreds to get a yes.
- ➤ Your first youth is a gift from Mother Nature; your second is a gift from yourself.
- ➤ Age doesn't make you forget—it teaches you what's important to remember.
- ➤ Wrinkles don't mean you're old; infants have plenty of them.
- ➤ Love is contagious. Go out and catch some.
- ➤ Never give up your dreams. They keep you awake.
- ➤ Youth isn't wasted on the young—or on anyone else.

The Least You Need to Know

- ➤ Distorted ideas about aging are all around you.
- ➤ Give up the idea that youth is problem-free.
- ➤ True youth comes from spirit. And spirit is ageless.
- ➤ Attitude affirmations are powerful ammunition against negative thinking.
- ➤ Hattietudes bring happiness.

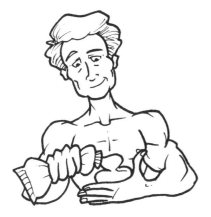

S = SKINCARE
Means Treating
It Right

Of the four E.A.S.E. steps for looking and feeling younger, our S—skincare—is the one aspect of reversing aging that produces the most striking results in the shortest amount of time. But this doesn't happen automatically; you have to work at it.

Sadly, it seems the only parts of our skin that get any care are the parts that show. And not much care at that. In a morning filled with preparations for the day ahead, we rush through our shower, shampoo our hair, and splash water on our faces. Men shave and women dab on makeup. Then we cover everything up with the most flattering or functional clothing we can find, and we're off.

It's as if skincare is a necessary evil to get over with as quickly as possible. Few people consider luxuriating in a tub or taking the time to give themselves an all-over massage with moisturizing lotion.

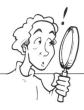

Our Skin Gets Short Shrift

Our lives have become too busy to give our skin the care it needs and deserves. We mostly view our skin as a covering and don't pay it much mind. It's a shame, too, because the skin is in fact the body's largest organ.

We must admit that we are delinquent in the care of our skin. Then what happens? Not only do we look old before our time, our general health suffers as well. Conversely, when we take care of our skin, it is reflected in every area of our lives.

What Is Skin?

The skin's surface is composed of cells, sebaceous glands, and sweat pores. It is covered with a thin layer of dead cells that are continually being pushed up to the surface. It's critical that these cells be removed, because if they remain on the body, they block the skin's capacity to breathe and eliminate wastes.

An acidic coating of oil protects the skin against bacteria. Under that are oil glands, blood vessels, nerves, and hair follicles, held together by a connective tissue called *collagen*. The condition of this collagen determines how wrinkled or lined your skin becomes through time or abuse.

Our First Defense

The skin is the body's first line of defense against toxic invaders that deplete the immune system. When our skin is healthy, it relieves stress, taking some of the burden off the liver, another of the body's major cleansing organs. If the liver is out of whack, its placement inside the body makes it difficult to pinpoint and treat.

Not so with the skin. Any problems show up immediately and give us the chance to take corrective action. It's hard to ignore signals from our skin.

Age Alert

If you're sick or under stress, your skin will appear dull and lifeless. You may also find that blemishes pop out and your color becomes pale and ashen, blotchy, or florid. If you have a cut that takes a long time to heal, consult your health care practitioner. This could be a sign of serious illness, such as diabetes. Healthy skin radiates wellness.

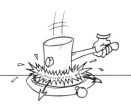

Time Stopper

The skin is a fabulous indicator of your health and well-being. Many things that are wrong with your health will show up on your skin. Train yourself to be acutely alert to its texture, tone, and quality. This awareness helps maintain a state of radiant health—and as a bonus, magnificent, youthful skin.

Great Skin Is in Your Hands

When we talk about *youthful skin,* we are in no way referring to adolescent skin, that oil-prone repository of acne, or even the skin of a newborn. We're talking about skin that has the potential to continuously revitalize. It will be toned and radiant with life only if it receives proper, ongoing care.

Don't take youth for granted. We want you to take how you age into your own hands and, where skincare is concerned, we mean this literally. You hands are your primary ally for keeping your skin looking and feeling young.

Young Skin = Young Body

When your skin is attractive, you feel attractive. It doesn't matter what shape it's in to begin with. Consistent care produces consistent results. Just don't give up—be relentless! It's worth it.

Exquisite skin is one of our most prized possessions. In fact, it is our birthright. When your skin is in good condition, your entire body looks and feels young. Perhaps you never considered that it is within your power to create beautiful, healthy skin for your entire life. It is.

Getting in Touch

Has it ever occurred to you that the places our bodies wrinkle the most are the very ones we've been cautioned not to touch?

We women are constantly told to be careful with our skin, especially the delicate skin around our eyes. How often have we heard that we must never scrub too vigorously, pull at the skin of our necks, or have very deep massages, lest we become bruised? We've been warned since childhood to be gentle and careful with our skin.

And what about how men treat their skin? Compared to what women are taught, men actually *abuse* it. They scrape their faces and necks with a razor every time they shave and, unless they're heavy smokers who spend every day of their lives in the sun, are none the worse for wear.

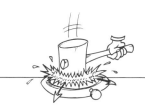

Time Stopper

Ponder this: How come wrinkles around men's eyes are called "character lines" and on women, "crow's-feet"? A little sexism, perhaps?

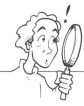

Age Alert

It's a little-known fact that what you put on the surface of the skin can be absorbed into the body. This applies equally to substances that are beneficial—like essential oils, vitamin creams—and those that are dangerous, like petroleum-based products. Don't think that because it's only on the surface it can't do real damage—or, on the positive side, provide real benefits.

What It Takes to Have Great Skin

It takes more than soap and water to have great skin. There are four essential elements to your program that will improve skin tone, texture, and elasticity:

➤ Exfoliation

➤ Circulation

➤ Hydration

➤ Detoxification

Exfoliation: Giving Your Skin the Brush

Exfoliation refers to expediting the shedding process in which dead cells flake away from the outer layer of the skin.

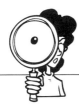

WatchWord

Webster's defines **exfoliation** as the casting off or coming off in flakes, scales, or layers, of skin, bark, etc.

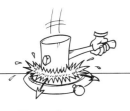

Time Stopper

An important reminder: When you purchase a brush for exfoliating your skin, make sure that the bristles are of natural fibers, not nylon or plastic. Use only when dry, never wet.

When we are children, we are growing so rapidly that this happens naturally, almost automatically. However, as we age, this slows down markedly, and we must take steps to facilitate this sloughing process.

By manually exfoliating with a dry brush each day, you can briskly remove the old skin. This unclogs pores and leaves a smooth, silky, blemish-free surface. With continuous exfoliation, you actually lighten age spots, smooth out imperfections, and prevent assorted irregularities that crop up.

Yes, those brown spots can be lightened and even disappear with assiduous dry brushing. For several years, Hattie lived in the Caribbean, where she baked in the sun without taking adequate precautions. Granted, it took *years* to correct, but with concentrated care, she was able to reverse the damage and erase the age spots that had formed on her skin. You can, too. Just keep working on it and be patient.

Daily brushing with a dry brush is a must if you want healthy, toned skin. Do this on each day *before* your shower or bath. It takes only five minutes to brush your skin vigorously from your shoulders to your feet. This removes dead cells and stimulates circulation.

One important reminder: Make sure the bristles are of natural fibers, not nylon, and use only when dry. Wetting makes the bristles too soft and allows the growth of bacteria, which can cause skin eruptions.

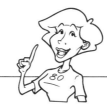

Voice of Experience

Licensed massage therapist Jim Graham says, "Massage is a tremendous complement to any program to slow the aging process. It helps feed the skin proper nutrition and improves circulation to speed recovery from the stress that ages our bodies."

Circulation: Getting Your Blood Flowing

Then there's circulation—the flow of blood through the veins, arteries, and capillaries. That's how we get nutrients and oxygen to our cells and get rid of impurities, wastes, and toxins. When our circulation is impaired, this nourishing/cleansing action is insufficient for our skin to be healthy.

Exfoliation provides surface stimulation, but it takes exercise and deep massage to guarantee abundant flow to every part of the body, inside and out.

Hydration: Keeping Your Cells Moist

The third component of skincare is hydration. Water, that precious fluid that carries youth-giving nutrients from our food into our tissues, is the single most important element in preventing cells from becoming dry and aged.

Hydration is achieved both externally and internally. Externally, our skin is moistened through long baths followed by the application of emollient-rich creams and lotions.

Everyone has heard about creams and lotions that are supposed to keep skin cells dewy and soft. While these external aids do assist in moisturizing the skin by plumping the cells with *humectants* and oils that prevent evaporation, we believe they aren't enough.

Internally, the hydration process is aided by what you put into your body. You have to take the inside track to truly keep your skin moist and supple. This involves supplying the skin with sufficient water (at least six to eight 8-ounce

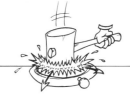

Time Stopper

Before showering, try the scratch test: Scratch the skin on your leg or forearm with your fingernails. If this leaves a trail of white lines, your skin is covered with dry, scaly cells. That tells you it's time to exfoliate and moisturize.

glasses per day) and consuming plenty of enzyme-rich raw fruits and freshly squeezed vegetable juices.

These high-powered nutrient-rich foods will moisturize your skin from within and prevent the breakdown and decay of tissues, which cause premature aging.

Detoxification: Getting Rid of Impurities

As our body's largest organ, our skin performs many functions that are vital for life. In addition to regulating body temperature, it is charged with the awesome task of nonstop removal of toxins through perspiration.

Cellular recycling is impeded when toxins accumulate in the body. These poisons may be from external sources, such as environmental pollution, or from internal forces, such as emotional stress, improper elimination of bodily wastes, or eating chemically laden foods.

The accumulation of these impurities speeds aging and saps the body of vitality.

Lotions and Potions and More

Almost any face cream or body cream on the market can make you *look* more youthful … temporarily.

What makes any skincare product work over the long term is its application. It's the consistent *touching*, not just the product, that makes the difference.

While costly products may contain extraordinarily beneficial ingredients, some relatively inexpensive creams also give excellent results.

Whatever you buy, make certain that it contains no mineral oils or petroleum products, ethyl or isopropyl alcohol, or artificial colors and scents. These ingredients, when absorbed by the skin, are carried into the systems of the body, where they have the potential of causing real harm.

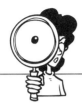

WatchWord

Humectants attract moisture to the skin's surface and hold it there. These moisturizing agents slow aging by making the skin softer and preventing dryness and chapping. Natural humectants include honey, which also has antibacterial properties, and aloe vera, which has natural healing properties.

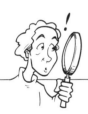

Age Alert

Beware of any antiperspirants or deodorants that contain aluminum or aluminum salts. They've been implicated in causing Alzheimer's disease, as well as some forms of cancer. The so-called deodorant stones, though "natural" aren't any safer as they contain aluminum salts. Also, the body needs to sweat. Perspiration is a vital way to eliminate poisons through the skin.

When considering products to combat the aging of the skin, explore *aromatherapy* oils. Using creams and lotions that contain aromatic essential oils from plants and flowers provides healing and beautifying nutrients to the skin. You can use these oils undiluted in the bath. If you apply them directly to the skin, however, they must be in diluted form.

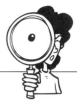

WatchWord

Detoxification is the thorough cleansing of toxins from the body. This is accomplished in three ways: perspiration, urination, and defecation.

Shedding Light on Sun Damage

In this age of holes in the earth's ozone layer, we shouldn't go out without protecting our skin from the sun. We'll not go into great detail about the effects of extensive exposure to the sun's rays. We've all been amply warned of the dangers of too much sun.

Ironically, widespread use of sunscreens is relatively new. Back in the 1960s, bottles of baby oil laced with iodine were as important as a new bikini when sunning on the beach or beside the pool.

Now we know that if you don't want your skin to look like a piece of thick, weathered cowhide, you've got to take protective measures. While you can still enjoy the sun's benefits, it's imperative that you use appropriate protection at all times and monitor your exposure carefully.

Don't fool yourself into thinking that the winter sun isn't damaging. There may be fewer daylight hours in December, but those rays are still powerful, so make sunscreen a skincare necessity for all seasons.

This caution is for men as well as for women, young as well as old. The sun is an equal-opportunity skin destroyer.

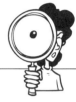

WatchWord

With the emerging awareness of holistic healing, the ancient practice of **aromatherapy** is finding its way into the mainstream. It uses the aromatic essential oils extracted from plants and flowers for both healing and cosmetic benefits. To be used safely, these volatile essences must be diluted in alcohol or nonessential oils. Though they are not soluble in water, they will impart their scent if used in a bath.

Make Your Skin Look Younger with Proper Care

These guidelines will help you develop a personal skincare regimen for younger and healthier-looking skin:

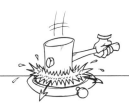

Time Stopper

You can still enjoy the benefits of the sun if you avoid exposure altogether from 11 A.M. to 3 P.M., when the sun is at its highest. Before and after these hours, wear a hat to protect your eyes, face, scalp and the oft-forgotten ears. Always, always use lots of sunscreen all over—including those tender tops of your feet.

➤ Make the four essentials of skincare—exfoliation, circulation, hydration, and detoxification—part of your daily routine. The more you do them, the more effective they will be.

➤ You've got to get rough to have smooth skin. Never let a day go by in which you are not rubbing, kneading, brushing, and briskly massaging your entire body. This includes your feet, hands, and scalp.

➤ The more circulation you stimulate, the more healthy and toned your skin becomes.

➤ There's nothing like a professional facial to thoroughly clean up your complexion. These pros have the special know-how, not to mention the tools that will give every pore a deep cleaning and leave your skin radiant. A good idea is to have a facial with each change of season— four times a year.

➤ Taking baths with aromatherapy oils will keep your skin supple and alleviate stress from your entire body.

➤ Never use petroleum jelly, mineral oil, baby oil, isopropyl alcohol, or any other substances on the skin that are not of the finest, natural, nonchemical, non-animal, cruelty-free ingredients.

➤ When choosing moisturizers, read the labels with care. Most commercial products contain petrochemicals and other synthetics that can cause dryness and block pores. Many are carcinogenic. For this reason, it's best to purchase skincare preparations, including sun blocks, at a natural-foods store.

➤ Keep all your nails groomed, particularly on your feet. Rub, buff, pumice all your calluses. If you ever develop a huge callus buildup, have it removed by a doctor. Don't let yourself grow a crust.

➤ To supplement your home care, consider having a professional manicure and pedicure. Dry, dead cuticles and calluses, particularly on your feet, are not only old-looking, they are also potentially painful. Anyone who has had sore feet knows what we mean. It's like having a toothache all over your body.

➤ Remember to scrub, buff, and oil your elbows. Wrinkly, dry elbows are a telltale sign of aging. You can even use extra-fine grain sandpaper to smooth them out. While you're at it, scrub and oil those knees, too.

➤ Try "talking" to your skin as you wash, oil, cream, and massage it. We all know how forceful thoughts can be. Positive messages and images have a powerful effect on the condition of your skin. Some affirming words to keep in mind: *nourish, moisturize, refine, tone, energize, stimulate, invigorate, regenerate, cleanse, soothe, smooth,* and *firm.* Add your own favorite words—qualities that will impact your consciousness.

The Least You Need to Know

➤ If you don't take care of your skin, it won't take care of you.

➤ The skin is not simply a covering. It is the body's largest organ.

➤ Exfoliation, circulation, hydration, and detoxification are the four main elements of skincare.

➤ We say you've got to get rough to get smooth.

➤ Protection from the sun becomes more crucial with each passing year.

➤ For yourself and the environment, choose only nonchemical, cruelty-free skincare products.

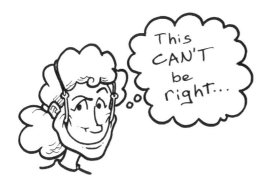

Chapter 15

Lift Your Face!

> ### In This Chapter
>
> ➤ BodyCheck of your face
>
> ➤ Facing your feelings about your face
>
> ➤ Skincare to reverse aging
>
> ➤ A young complexion starts on the inside
>
> ➤ Exercises for a youthful face

No matter what you look like, your face is your most identifying feature.

For many of us, it is also one of the most noticeable places we age. Unlike the rest of the body, there's no way to fully protect it. Even sunscreens and big hats can't foil sun and environmental damage. This type of damage affects us at any age, young or old.

Life Shows Up on Our Faces

Indulgences, like drinking and smoking, also leave their marks, etching wrinkles about our mouths and eyes. Vestiges of work and worry, as well as the foods we eat, are imprinted there, too.

These Lift Your Face™ exercises, along with the skincare recommendations you learned in the previous chapter, go a long way in reversing the damage that causes aging of the face.

Does this mean you will never have a line or wrinkle? Of course not. It would be unfair and untrue to promise this. But what we *do* promise is that you have within you the power to create a glowing, more youthful face, no matter what you've heard to the contrary.

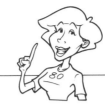

Voice of Experience

Legendary beauty Audrey Hepburn expressed herself so eloquently on the subject of appearance: "The beauty of a woman is not in a facial mole, but true beauty in a woman is reflected in her soul."

Facing Your Face

By now, you've probably realized that the most effective way to confront aging is to stare it, ahem, right in the face. Pun definitely intended.

As you did in Chapter 2, "How Old Does Your Skin Look?" when we asked you to do a BodyCheck of your skin, we want you to inspect your face thoroughly. Make note of all indications of aging: sagging jowls, droopy eyelids, puffiness, double chins, enlarged pores, wrinkles, lines, spots, growths … anything you see that you'd like to improve.

BodyCheck of the Face

In front of a brightly lit mirror, examine your face. Mark what you see on the illustration. Write a description in the column beside it.

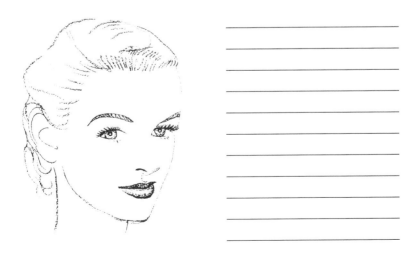

Now that you've looked at your face this carefully, you may be discouraged, if not absolutely revolted. Take heart: The first step to any change is acknowledging what bothers you.

Clearly you saw many things about your face that you like and even love, and we want to give them attention as well. Focusing only on the negative, while helpful in initiating change, can be daunting. Acknowledging our positive features gives us confidence to tackle what we dislike.

There's Lots to Love

As we age, we tend to focus on the downside. Let's turn that around. The first part of this next exercise asks you to list all the wonderful things you see about your face. Some things are obvious (your long eyelashes or powerful jaw line, for example), but others are more subtle, like your delicate earlobes or dimples.

What I Love About My Face

List 10 characteristics about your face that please you.

1. _____
2. _____
3. _____
4. _____
5. _____
6. _____
7. _____
8. _____
9. _____
10. _____

Taking Your Face in Hand

If we believed what our mothers and the cosmetics industry tell us, we'd handle our faces with kid gloves and sit back and wait for the wrinkles to come as we save our money for a face-lift.

Wrong.

Has it ever occurred to you that the places where your body wrinkles the most readily are the very ones you've been told not to touch? We are constantly cautioned to be careful with the delicate skin around our eyes, and to be careful with the skin on our neck. Conventional advice is that you should never pull at the skin on your face.

Don't push at it, either.

Wrong again.

We will explode those common myths ("Be gentle …" "Be careful …" "Never pull the skin around your eyes …") … all those don'ts that leave us afraid to do anything but wash with lukewarm water and gently pat dry.

Our methods for caring for the face might seem radical, but they are completely safe and produce extraordinary results. Long-lasting, too.

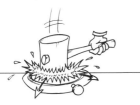

Time Stopper

As we age, our circulation becomes more sluggish, especially where blood vessels are tiny, as in the face. To encourage blood flow, massage your face vigorously; don't just dab at it when you wash and cream your face. Make sure that you also include the neck in this ritual. It needs all the attention it can get.

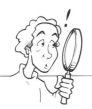

Age Alert

Beware: Don't use synthetic bristle brushes and nylon puffs on your face and neck. Stay away from loofa sponges, too, even though they're natural. All three can be damaging, because they tend to be too scratchy. Loofas also collect bacteria like crazy.

At first, these recommendations may seem shocking. You may even say, "No way! You're telling me to *stretch* my skin. That'll make me look worse, not better."

Giving Your Face the Brush

As with the rest of your body, the skin on your face and neck needs to be exfoliated to stay young and soft. Daily dry brushing is the best way to do this.

Our favorite facial brush technically isn't even a brush at all. It's a soft rubber cat groomer, with pliant bristle-like fingers on both sides. About three inches long and an inch and a half wide, this tool is firm enough to provide a good massage, yet soft enough not to damage delicate facial tissue or blood vessels that are so close to the surface. Also, it's quite inexpensive and seems to last forever.

If this rubber cat groomer doesn't appeal to you, a soft-bristle brush made of natural fibers also works. Anything else can do damage, especially since you'll be working so deeply.

Here's the best way to brush:

➤ Using your clean, dry brush, rub upward and out in a circular motion on each cheek, applying pressure to the bone. Then brush your chin, forehead, and neck.

Note: You must use a *dry* brush for this process. This not only sloughs off dead skin cells, it also unclogs pores and increases circulation.

➤ Using tepid water and a natural cleanser, wash and rinse your face to remove dead skin cells dislodged by brushing. Rub dry with a clean towel, preferably white.

It Doesn't Happen Overnight

Immediately, you will notice that your skin has a rosy glow. Brushing has stimulated the blood flow, and this increased circulation gives you heightened color and improved texture and tone. But the lines, wrinkles, and age spots are still there. Is there no hope?

Yes. It just takes longer. Sometimes much, much longer.

Those lines, wrinkles, and age spots didn't just show up one day. They took years to develop, and they aren't going to disappear overnight. Naturally, we all want quick results. We wish we could promise them to you in every instance. But the deeper the problem, the longer it takes to correct. For example, it took Hattie a full two years to repair sun damage on her face. The good side is that within those two years, her skin could have been aging more. It didn't. Her persistence paid off. Yours will, too.

Rubbing It In

Also integral to creating a younger-looking face is massage.

Since blood carries food and oxygen throughout the body and takes away impurities, wastes, and toxins, proper circulation is essential for radiant, healthy skin.

Because of its location (at the top of the body) and its construction (bone just under the skin), the head—and consequently, the face—is often short-changed.

Beside headstands, one of the best ways to bring fresh blood to the tissues of the face is massage. It stimulates the skin and all underlying layers of muscle and fatty tissue and assists in the regenerative process. This revitalizes musculature and increases skin tone.

How to Massage Your Face

You may have been warned that rubbing your face and pulling at your skin will make it sag. To that we say "Ha!"

In fact, the only way to keep your facial skin toned and, consequently, youthful, is to provide it with

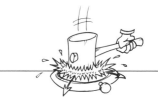

Time Stopper

If you want your skin to stay young forever, you have to work at it every single day. Daily skin brushing is for your entire life.

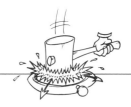

Time Stopper

When using oil for skincare or massage, only use a little at a time. Decant what you need into a smaller bottle, or pour what you will be using into a bowl and refrigerate the rest. Unrefrigerated oils become rancid, even if you can't smell it, and cause free-radical damage. This results in premature aging.

153

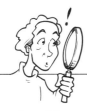

Age Alert

Great skin is more than skin deep. No cream can take the place of proper nutrition, and no makeup can cover the effects of improper nutrition.

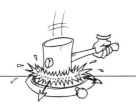

Time Stopper

We've been warned to avoid oily food, lest we get fat. But eliminating oily foods starves our skin. It makes no sense to put expensive creams on the surface of the skin when you aren't feeding it from within. Don't avoid avocados, olives, and nuts because of their high fat content. Eat them as part of a balanced, healthy diet, and you won't gain weight. What you will gain is a radiant glow.

deep, vigorous stimulation. That's where these massage techniques come in. Here goes:

1. Prepare your face by applying a light coat of oil or cream. Believe it or not, the best oils won't be found in the skincare departments of most drug or specialty stores. You have to visit your neighborhood health shop and look in the food department. What you want to buy is one of the unrefined, cold-pressed oils—preferably organic. Almond, olive, and avocado are winners.

2. Pinch the entire face and neck between your thumb and forefinger, quickly pressing and releasing to keep the skin pliable and elastic.

3. Using your knuckles, start at the chin and massage deeply in small outward circles until you reach your cheekbones. Don't focus on lifting the skin. The effectiveness of this massage comes from pressing forcefully into the bones.

4. If, after this massage, you feel your skin is oily, rinse off the excess and dry with a clean towel.

The Inside Story

While exfoliation and massage increase circulation to the face, your diet has a lot to say about the condition of your complexion.

Eating carefully selected, enzyme-rich, antioxidant foods will guarantee that the skin is well-fed from within. It takes at least three to five servings of fresh, raw fruits and vegetables a day to properly nourish the skin from within. Notice we said *raw* fruits and vegetables. Uncooked foods provide necessary enzymes that are destroyed by heat.

Of special help to the skin are foods rich in beta-carotene—the dark yellow and orange fruits and veggies. This includes carrots, sweet potatoes, winter squashes, pumpkins, mangos, apricots, papayas, and cantaloupes. Citrus fruits as well as tomatoes, are rich in vitamin C, which aids in regeneration.

In tandem with a diet rich in nutrients, the body requires adequate hydration. You need to drink six to eight 8-ounce glasses of water a day to moisturize the skin.

In addition, copious amounts of green tea—either hot or cold—and freshly squeezed fruit and vegetable juices should be included in each day's regimen. Try never to go a day without one freshly squeezed juice.

Exercise Your Face for Youth

Going along with the old adage that until you are 30 you have the face that nature gave you, but after that, you have the face you deserve, these Lift Your Face exercises help you "deserve" a great face.

Jim Carrey and Marcel Marceau will have nothing on you as you bite your tongue, pull your ears, and blow up your cheeks like Dizzy Gillespie—all to develop strong, supple facial muscles that radiate youth.

You may take your body to the gym, but what are you doing—besides eating and talking— to give your face a workout?

With Lift Your Face, you will focus on the underlying tissues and pay particular attention to the musculature around your mouth, neck, and shoulders, where the body holds considerable stress. This stress contributes to wrinkling.

Unlike any other exercises that profess to tone the face and neck, these are the only ones that deal with the muscles *inside* the mouth. Wrinkles that appear on the face often stem from tightness in the underlying muscle tissue.

Lift Your Face—Exercises for the Face

Do these exercises when you wash your face in the morning and at bedtime to discourage development of vertical creases between your nose and mouth and to develop strong cheek muscles. You will feel this working the cheek muscles located inside your mouth.

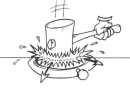

Time Stopper

Before you begin these Lift Your Face exercises, remember to wash your hands. You will be sticking your fingers in your mouth.

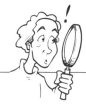

Age Alert

The best thing about these facial exercises is that you don't have to go anyplace, use any special equipment, or even budget time and money to do them. A study conducted by the Southwest Health Institute in Phoenix, Arizona, shows that 75 percent of morning exercisers are likely to still be at it one year later, as opposed to 50 percent of midday exercisers and 25 percent of those who work out in the evening. Could it be that, as the day progresses, we think up more excuses to avoid working out?

Push-Ups for the Cheeks

This exercise, push-ups for the cheeks, will help soften those deep vertical creases—those "marionette lines"—between the nose and lips.

1. Stand up straight in front of the mirror, keeping your shoulders relaxed.

2. Open your mouth wide. Pull your lips tightly over your teeth so that you look like you have no teeth.

3. Now firmly press the knuckles of each hand against each cheekbone and feel your muscles flex to iron out the lines. Continue pressing hands into cheeks as you stretch your mouth open wide and say "Ahh."

4. Then purse your lips together and say "Ooh."

5. Continue to contract and relax your lips, saying "Ah" and "Ooh."

Repetitions: 50

Push-ups for the cheeks.

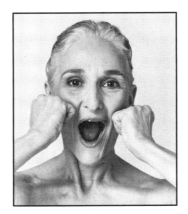 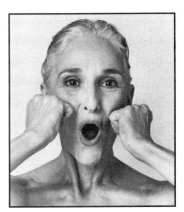

Blow-Ups

Another of my favorite cheek exercises is called blow-ups:

1. Keeping your mouth firmly closed, blow up your cheeks in puffs like inflating a tire with a pump.

2. Hold for a count of 10.

3. Release.

Repetitions: 10

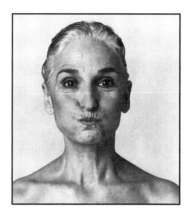

Blow-ups.

Tongue-in-Cheek

A terrific way to soften your expression and remove wrinkles and frown lines around your mouth is the tongue-in-cheek exercise:

1. Push your tongue firmly against each cheek.

2. Continue pressing your tongue against the inside of your mouth, working around your lips.

3. Continue pressing outward to stretch tight areas around the mouth and cheeks.

Repetitions: 5

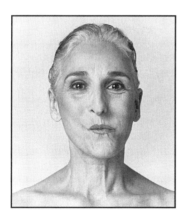 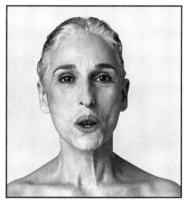

Tongue-in-cheek.

The Rubber Band

Because of all the talking and eating we do in a lifetime, the muscles surrounding the lips carry a lot of tension—and get very little attention. One of the hallmarks of aging is the appearance of creases around the mouth. This exercise will correct or prevent that problem.

157

1. Hold your mouth partly open with your forefingers; pull the corners apart as wide as possible.

2. Quickly remove your fingers and let your mouth "snap" back to its relaxed position.

3. Open your mouth wide. With your thumb and forefinger, rapidly pinch and release your lips all around your mouth.

4. Work your way all around the upper and lower lips and move into your cheeks, paying extra attention to the cheeks.

Repetitions: 5

The rubber band.

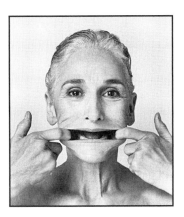

Bite Your Tongue

The tongue, interestingly, happens to be the strongest muscle in the body. No one ever thinks of actually exercising it other than when we talk or eat ... or kiss!

1. Open the mouth wide and stick your tongue out as far as it will go.

2. Flatten and widen your tongue, and hold it there for a count of 10; then pull it back.

3. Lightly bite your tongue at random.

4. Stick out your tongue and close your lips lightly around it.

5. Then blow hard and make that obnoxious noise your mother told you not to.

Repetitions: 3

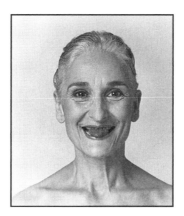

Bite your tongue.

For Your Neck

Our necks age more quickly than our faces because we touch them less. This exercise increases circulation *and* gets rid of wrinkled skin. It's especially helpful in fighting double chins.

1. Hold your head erect and shoulders relaxed.
2. Grab the skin on your neck with your thumb and forefingers and randomly pinch and pull it.

Repetitions: 25

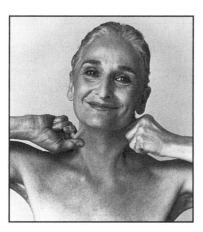

For your neck.

159

Are You Pulling My Ear?

One common sign of aging that you never may have considered is droopy, dry earlobes. This exercise is great for circulation.

1. Give your earlobes a mini-workout by massaging them with skin-softening lotion or oil.

2. Grasping your earlobes with your thumb and forefinger, pull them down. Pinch, twist, and wiggle them around.

Repetitions: 25

Are you pulling my ear?

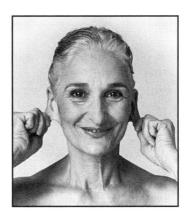

The Least You Need to Know

➤ Awareness of how your face has aged helps you take steps to change how it is aging.

➤ Loving your face supports your age–reversing efforts.

➤ To have a great complexion, you must brush and massage your skin daily.

➤ It can take years to take years off your face.

➤ Give your face a lift with Lift Your Face exercises.

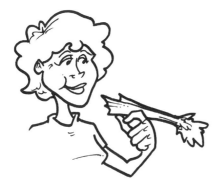

Chapter 16

E = EATING—It's a Weighty Matter

In This Chapter

➤ Is "ideal weight" ideal?

➤ Calculating weight for your height and frame

➤ About calories and weight control

➤ How exercise burns calories

➤ Taking time to eat

The final E in E.A.S.E.—Eating—is so important that we need more than this one chapter to cover it for you. The entire next section—Part 4, "Putting Youth on Your Plate"—is devoted to a way of eating that will radically alter how you eat for life.

For now, we'll just concentrate on the question of weight.

Changes for a Lifetime

Although simple changes in Exercise, Attitude, and Skincare provide noticeable results right from the start, it takes far more than upping your activity level, shifting your mindset, or dry brushing your skin to break a lifetime of deeply ingrained eating habits that age you. To do this, it's important to explore your feelings about weight.

What's Your Ideal Weight?

How's that for a loaded question?

The term "ideal weight" would seem to indicate that there is a specific number on a scale that is perfect for every age and every stage.

This couldn't be farther from the truth. In fact, preoccupation with this number almost guarantees that you'll be unable to reach a goal that's realistic, desirable, and healthy.

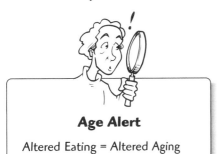

Age Alert

Altered Eating = Altered Aging

Of greater importance than setting a hard-and-fast weight goal is feeling comfortable and happy with your size. That way, you won't be obsessed with your weight. This does not give you license to eat yourself into a stupor or resign yourself to a lifetime of obesity. We're reinforcing a sense of self-respect that causes you to feel good about yourself, even if your body doesn't look exactly like you want it to. Often when the pressure to be thin is replaced by self-acceptance and self-love, losing weight becomes easier.

But Is It Realistic?

Occasionally, a person chooses an "ideal" weight that is in line with realistic goals that they feel they can achieve.

But this is rare.

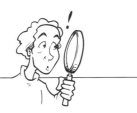

Age Alert

Don't weigh yourself every day. Very often, if you see that you've lost weight, you'll eat more to celebrate. And, if you see that you've gained weight, you'll eat more out of frustration. Either way, the scale wins.

Too often the opposite is true. Whether it's from a goal weight on a chart in a doctor's office or the pages of fashion magazines, most people have such unrealistic expectations that they never reach the weight they desire. Often, if they do, they are so anxious that they are unable to stay there long enough to enjoy being there.

How sad it is for so many people to feel like failures in the weight-loss department. Let's break that pattern.

Don't Get Stuck on the Numbers

This fixation on a number sets up a dangerous yo-yo pattern of weight loss and gain that jeopardizes your physical health.

It's no surprise that most people who adhere to stringent weight-reduction programs often lose weight; however, as soon as they reach their target number, they go off the diet. What happens then? As soon as they resume their former eating habits, the weight returns. Then they starve themselves back to that magic number on the scale.

The yo-yo is in motion.

Not only does their weight go up and down, their mood does, too.

Yo-yo dieters have lost sight of the big picture. While some weight fluctuations can be normal and healthy, those caused by serial dieting are neither normal nor healthy.

Even more drastic, not to mention more dangerous, is what we call the *starve-and-stuff syndrome*. This is a pattern of severely restrictive dieting (starving), followed by periods of eating inordinate amounts of food (stuffing). Very often, people want to stay in starvation mode, as is the case with anorexics, but the body's need for nourishment overrides their determination.

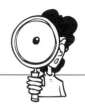

WatchWord

The **starve-and-stuff syndrome** is a term we coined to describe the pattern of severely restrictive dieting to lose weight (starving), followed by periods of rapid weight gain from massive overeating (stuffing).

Are You What You Weigh?

At different times, as life circumstances change, weight fluctuates. This is usually five to eight pounds in either direction and should not be cause for concern.

If you're obsessed with weight and conscious of every ounce you put on, you are setting yourself up for disappointment and, ultimately, failure. Nothing can make you hungrier than constantly worrying about what you've eaten and if you've gained any weight.

As much as we know that weight should not be the measure of a person's worth, too often we judge others by what they weigh. We make the same value judgments about ourselves, too.

Putting these judgments aside, there is considerable health value in maintaining a weight that suits your height, body type, and lifestyle. The trick is to determine what feels right for you and to resist being hung up on an image that is virtually impossible to maintain.

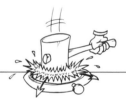

Time Stopper

When setting your weight-loss goals, be realistic about how much weight you need to lose and how long it will take you to lose it. Remember: You didn't gain that extra 45 pounds overnight, or even during the past week. You certainly won't lose that weight overnight, or even in a week or 10 days.

For realistic weight loss that won't come bouncing back in a matter of weeks, expect to lose one to two pounds a week. This way, loss is slow but sure.

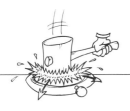

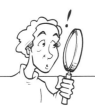

Remember: You are not what you weigh. You are a unique individual with certain attributes and certain liabilities. When you "weigh" your value as a human being, don't use a scale.

Weights and Measures

We're familiar with those height and weight charts proposed by insurance companies and health care professionals, but few of us know how these figures are computed. Here's their formula:

➤ To determine the recommended weight for women: Allow 100 pounds for the first five feet of height, and add five pounds for each additional inch.

➤ For men, start with 106 pounds for the initial five feet, and add six pounds per additional inch.

For instance, for a woman who is five feet, seven inches tall and has a medium frame, the weight is 135; for a six-foot man of medium frame, it is 178.

What Frame Size Are You?

Allow for five to eight pounds less if you have a small frame; five to eight pounds more if your frame is large. Note: One way to determine the size of your frame or bone structure is to wrap the fingers of your left hand around your right wrist. If your thumb and middle finger overlap, your frame is small; if they meet, it's medium; if there is a space, it's large.

Burning Those Calories

What we weigh is determined not just by how much we eat, but by the kind of food we consume and our body's ability to metabolize or burn this food.

When your body weight is exactly what you want it to be, you have found the balance between food intake and energy output.

This energy output is measured in terms of *calories* (actually, kilocalories) burned.

How Many Calories Are There in a Pound?

Three-thousand-five-hundred calories go into one pound of fat. That's 3,500 calories entering the body as food or being burned up through exercise.

Calories in, Calories Out

Because body weight obeys the fundamental laws of thermodynamics (calories consumed versus calories burned), weight loss occurs when the body burns more calories than it consumes.

For this reason, calorie-counting became a reliable means of weight management for many people. Unfortunately, it becomes too time-consuming and distracting to have to calculate the number of calories in certain foods or serving sizes. Everyone knows that if it's not easy, we'll probably give it up. Most people do.

Doing the Math

Here's how to determine how many calories per day your body needs to maintain a specific weight:

➤ Multiply your desired body weight by 10 calories per pound. Use this figure as your baseline.

➤ To this baseline, add three calories per pound of desired weight if you are a sedentary person; five calories per pound if you are moderately active; and 10 calories per pound if you regularly exercise at a strenuous level.

➤ The sum of these numbers is the total number of calories your body needs per day to maintain your desired body weight. If you consume more calories than this without increasing your exercise level, your weight will increase.

Using these figures, our five-foot, seven-inch woman whose target weight is 135 would need approximately 1,755 calories per day to maintain her

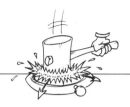

Time Stopper

If you normally relax in front of the TV or by playing bridge, up your activity level by choosing fun activities that involve movement: dancing, playing miniature golf, swimming, going bowling— anything active. The maximum number of calories you can burn during an hour of card playing is 95, whereas waltzing can whirl away 195 to 205 an hour. An hour of square-dancing promenades and do-si-dos burns between 330 and 510 calories. Also, it's harder to eat when you're dancing than it is when you're playing cards!

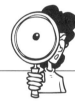

WatchWord

The technical definition of **calorie** is the amount of heat needed to raise the temperature of one gram of water one degree Centigrade. It is the unit for measuring the energy produced by food when it is oxidized in the body.

165

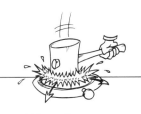

Time Stopper

If you've ever doubted the power of aerobics to burn calories, listen to this: Aerobic exercise, such as swimming, biking, and rapid walking, speeds up your metabolism for as long as four to eight hours *after* you stop. How great! Your body will keep burning calories long after you've finished your workout.

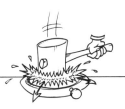

Time Stopper

Be honest about how much exercise you do. You may think you are strenuously active, but unless you are an Olympic athlete, you work out in the gym for several hours a day, or possibly, you're the parent of three preschoolers, you are probably only moderately active at best. If the truth be told, most of us lead sedentary lives.

weight at 135. Since she weighs more than that, she is obviously eating too much. The only way for her to effectively lose weight is to reduce her caloric intake and add a program of exercise as vigorous as she can manage.

Let Someone Else Do the Counting

If you'd rather not do the calorie-counting yourself, you might consider a diet plan that does it for you.

The successful food programs offer plans without even mentioning calories. They speak about portions or serving sizes and categories. Nevertheless, these plans are based on carefully calculated caloric controls, even if they don't talk about it. They've done the legwork and have given us complete plans that are easy to follow.

Many people find group programs effective and even enjoyable. Self-discipline is easier when you have backup support.

Choosing Calories Wisely

As a rule, calories are measured in grams, not ounces or pounds. We're talking *small*. A gram weighs only 0.0353 of an ounce.

To eat healthily, watch where your calories come from. Most available energy comes from three major food categories:

➤ Carbohydrates, which contain four calories per gram

➤ Proteins, also four calories per gram

➤ Fats, a whopping nine calories per gram

Bear this in mind. The calories in soft drinks and junk foods are calculated in exactly the same way as the calories in whole-grain bread and nutritious foods. It's not just the number of calories you're after, but the nutritive value of the food as well.

A Piece of Cake?

Who do you know who will eat a piece of cake and a chocolate bar to satisfy food cravings and then skip meals because they've used up their day's calorie allowance? They may stay enviably thin, but at the expense of their health. Not a great bargain. In time, this catches up with them in the form of sickness and low vitality.

Don't squander your day's calorie quota on foods that will do more harm than good. You'll only age faster. Almost nothing is more aging than being malnourished year in and year out.

One of Hattie's clients, an attractive professional woman in her 50s had been virtually starving herself to keep thin. For most of her life, she had unlimited energy, and when she felt at all tired, she'd grab a candy bar for a boost. After several years of eating this way, she became chronically fatigued to the point that she could barely put in a day's work.

"It took so much convincing to get her to eat nutritious food instead of fast chocolate snacks," Hattie recalls. "She practically had to be force-fed. I introduced her to whole grains, nuts, avocados, organic eggs—all foods she avoided because she feared they would make her fat."

After years of avoiding healthy food, she was quite surprised to learn that it was delicious. Not only did she not gain weight, but her energy and zest for life were restored.

Time Stopper

You can enjoy a large bowl of pasta primavera, full of high-energy pasta and steamed fresh vegetables, and a salad on the side, and feel totally satisfied—and with far fewer calories than a small, cholesterol-laden cheeseburger with lettuce, tomato, and mayonnaise, and a side of fries.

Teach Yourself to Slow Down

Fast food is one thing. Fast eating is quite another.

By eating slowly and chewing your food thoroughly, you give your stomach time to send signals to your brain that you are no longer hungry. Here are some sure-fire slowdown techniques:

➤ Turn the TV set off and the answering machine on, with the volume turned off.

➤ Put your fork down between bites.

➤ Don't pick up another bite of food until you have chewed and swallowed the food in your mouth.

➤ If you're eating alone, step away from the table for a few minutes—five would be great—before returning to your meal.

➤ When dining with friends, take a rest between courses or midway through your meal. Just put your fork down and talk with your companions.

➤ Pace yourself. Try being the last person to finish each course.

➤ Never wait less than 30 minutes to give your brain time to pick up the signals from your tummy that you've had enough to eat. Besides, you're much more likely to get indigestion if you eat too quickly. That certainly takes the joy out of eating.

The Least You Need to Know

➤ There is no ideal weight that is appropriate for everybody.

➤ Calorie-counting is a reliable tool of weight management.

➤ You can eat more without gaining weight if you increase the amount you exercise.

➤ Don't skip meals to make up for eating high-calorie snacks.

➤ It's usually easier to stick to a weight-loss program if you join a group.

➤ Eating too rapidly hampers digestion and leaves you feeling heavy and exhausted.

Part 4

Putting Youth on Your Plate

Certainly exercise, attitude, and skincare are vital to staying young, but we believe that unless we supply our bodies with powerful nutrients, we will be unable to sustain the level of health necessary for a life of youth. Thus, the final E in our E.A.S.E. program—EATING—warrants special attention.

No one would deny the importance of proper eating. We're reminded of it constantly. The connection between aging and eating, however, has not been emphasized strongly enough. That's why we've devoted an entire part of the book to this, not just a chapter.

Most people think of a diet as a short-term change in their eating pattern that will produce rapid results. Not us! We want you to alter how you eat for your entire life so that effective results keep coming. We debunk many commonly held food myths and supply you with a completely new way to think about eating for youth. Added to this are great suggestions for vitamins, minerals, and other powerful supplements to give your body the raw materials to sustain health and youth.

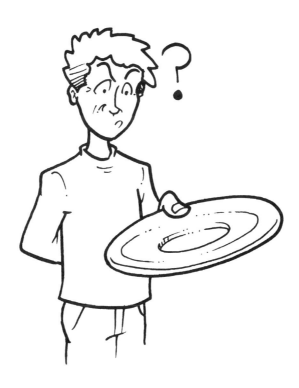

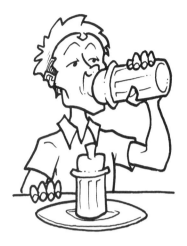

Chapter 17

You're as Young as You Eat

In This Chapter

➤ Changing your lifetime eating habits

➤ Satisfying your appetite

➤ Learning what foods you eat may be hazardous to your health

➤ Substituting "youth-foods" for "nonfoods"

➤ Busting food myths that rob you of youth

It's shocking how little understanding people have about the relationship between food and aging. Even esteemed professionals espouse vastly contradictory opinions, leaving many people confused and misinformed. We want you to totally give up the concept of DIET—be it for weight loss or for maintaining youth.

Changing Lifetime Habits

To eat for youth, you must transform *how* and *what* you eat for your entire life. Though it often takes years for the benefits of enduring age reversal to show up, you will start looking and feeling younger as soon as you start making changes.

We all know how difficult it is to change habits, particularly those that have been around for most of our lives.

What makes changing our food habits especially challenging is that the media continuously tempts us with images of sizzling steaks surrounded by mountains of mashed potatoes holding lakes of gravy and dazzling pictures of hillocks of ice cream drizzled with chocolate and caramel sauces.

Who can resist this visual orgy? But resist we must, if we want to achieve lifetime youth.

It's Got to Taste Great

To be healthy and youthful forever means permanently changing how you eat, not just until you drop a few pounds or look a certain way.

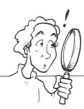

Age Alert

You didn't develop your eating habits overnight, or even over the last month. It takes time to change the eating habits of a lifetime. Be patient, and be kind to yourself.

Food is life and life is food. You shouldn't feel guilty about your appetite, cravings, and desires. These are natural and desirable human attributes, not frailties.

If you're going to stick with a program for a lifetime, it had better include plenty of food that you love. If your food isn't truly delicious and satisfying, you'll ultimately revert to your former eating style.

Says Hattie, "What's the point of living a long life if you can't eat the foods you love? I found foods I love that love me, and I enjoy every bite of every meal. Even though I had to learn to say no to some of my all-time favorites, it wasn't a hardship, because I learned how to choose so many new and tasty foods that I am completely satisfied."

What You Eat May Be Aging You

When we are young, we tend to think of food in terms of pleasing our appetites and whether or not it will make us fat. Then, with time and maturity, our awareness expands to include how what we eat makes us feel.

Usually we don't pay too much attention to the correlation between food and health until something goes wrong.

It's only recently that the connection between improper eating and premature aging has received attention. We want you to acknowledge this connection and keep it uppermost in your mind. When you focus on how improper eating ages you, your self-discipline will improve markedly.

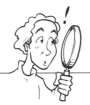

Age Alert

The active ingredient in most cola drinks is phosphoric acid. Its pH is 2.8, and it will dissolve a nail in about four days. Some people pour it over their car battery terminals to bubble away the corrosion and use it to loosen rusted bolts. And we drink this?

French Fries, Anyone?

There are certain foods that, no matter how great we think they taste, are disastrous to our health. The friendly French fry tops this list.

Ice cream runs a close second. And so does pizza ... and those carbonated cola drinks.

No sane person would claim that these qualify as healthy by any stretch of the imagination, yet millions of people eat these foods every day without a second thought. They taste good, they're fast, and they're usually just a drive-thru away. Some even advertise their nutritional values to lure us into believing that they are actually good for us.

Have you ever heard that pizza is the perfect food? For Madison Avenue, perhaps, but not for your health. It's a wonder that the high-gluten flour crust, combined with high-fat, gummy overcooked cheese and salty sauce, is even digestible.

When Foods Are Really Harmful

If you're serious about looking and feeling younger, be prepared to ignore the hype and the sizzle of these popular foods and banish them from your diet. "Banish" is a pretty strong word, but that's exactly what we're advising you to do.

To put it straight: Certain foods are hazardous to your health and are making you sick and old before your time. In this chapter, you'll learn what they are and how to avoid them.

> **Time Stopper**
>
> Just say no. It's perfectly acceptable to say "None for me, thanks" when someone offers you unhealthy foods. You can even say "No thanks, I'm eating for youth now."

Some Foods Are "Nonfoods"

Unfortunately, just recognizing that something is unhealthy is not enough to keep it off your plate. We need much stronger motivation. Without a specific plan of attack to keep us on target, we will inadvertently slip back into sloppy eating.

It's hard to deny ourselves the goodies and comfort foods. But it's worth it.

In the RetroAge Eating Program, Hattie decided it would be a good idea to distinguish foods that are unhealthy or aging from those that generate youth and health.

To help you master this style of eating, we have created two categories:

➤ **"Nonfoods."** Anything that is commonly regarded as food, but doesn't foster health.

➤ **"Youth-foods."** Foods that nourish the body without triggering binges or mood-swings.

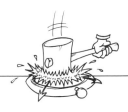

Time Stopper

Positive feedback pays off. Give yourself points for what you *don't* do, not just for what you do. For example, if you eat only half a piece of pecan pie, acknowledge yourself for not eating the whole thing. If you ride your exercise bike for only 15 minutes instead of the 30 you had intended, thank yourself for the 15 minutes you did ride. Remember to work for progress, not perfection.

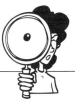

WatchWord

We use the term **nonfoods** to describe whatever we take into our bodies that is commonly termed "food" but is nutritionally deficient or even deleterious to our health. The term **youth-foods** describes those items that enhance the health of our body and foster youth.

It's easier for us to stay on target if we have terms to help keep us focussed.

These distinctions give us something concrete to hold on to. Every time someone suggests going out for burgers and fries, the word nonfoods will flash into your consciousness and remind you to select something else, hopefully, a youth-food.

Please don't think of us as the Food Police who're out to arrest anyone who eats anything we deem unhealthy. We assure you that our intent is to guide you to eat foods that create youth, which is what we all desire.

You Can't Stop Eating, but You Can Give Up Nonfoods

This is the rationale behind using the term "nonfoods":

➤ Some foods are as addictive as alcohol and drugs.

➤ People can successfully break the hold alcohol and drugs have on them by cutting them completely out of their lives.

➤ It is impossible to completely avoid food.

➤ So, to break the attachment to unhealthy foods, we designate them as nonfoods.

That way, we can work toward giving them up 100 percent.

Facing the Devil

We want to make it clear that when we use the term "nonfoods," we're not referring to the shelves of inedible things, like paper towels and detergents, that your cashier scans as a nonfood. We're referring to specific food products that deprive our bodies of health: sugared cereals, processed meats such as hot dogs, artificial sweeteners, sodas, cookies, candies, cakes, white flour, white sugar, white rice, and even white pasta.

174

To be called "youth-foods," they must be fresh and whole, as close to their natural state as possible. And if you can buy organically grown and pesticide-free products, that's even better.

For successful age-reversing, systematically elimi-nate all nonfoods from your diet, no matter how difficult it is or how long it takes.

It Never Ends

There's almost nothing more difficult than resist-ing all the unhealthy foods that call to us every day. It's impossible to pass a restaurant or grocery store, or even to go to a friend's house, without being tempted by these seductively delicious-looking deadly foods.

They're everywhere.

Use the words—nonfoods and youth-foods—as a constant reminder to weed out everything un-healthy from your diet. While you may never be able to eliminate them completely, this distinction will empower you to eat less and less of them.

Regrettably, the temptation never goes away. You'll have to muster all your self-discipline—as well as your survival instincts—to resist them. We know. We too are faced with the same temptations as you are, but we keep working to avoid them.

The bonus is, the more you are able to resist, the healthier and younger you will be. And that's a promise. It has worked for us; it can work for you.

Breaking Free of the Myths That Age Us

Now it's time to blitz outdated nutritional con-cepts and commonly held myths about eating.

You may find some of these subjects shocking. They certainly contradict concepts many of us have held for years. All we ask is that you read on with an open mind.

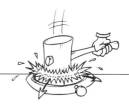

Time Stopper

Make age-reversal a family proj-ect. Call a family meeting to dis-cuss each member's health and well-being. Then set up health goals for everyone—mom, dad, and even the children, if they're still at home. You might even want to make a chart to reflect these goals. This is an especially effective technique to use if someone in the family is over-weight, or if a family member has health issues. This takes the focus off that individual and makes it a family project.

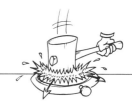

Time Stopper

Just as fire can warm us in the winter or cook our meals, it can burn our homes and woodlands. The same goes for food. It only becomes a problem when it is abused or misused.

We'll be tackling one myth after another. The great thing about this is that you can connect to them and start implementing changes in your own way of eating. With each change, you'll begin to experience immediate positive results. This encourages you to continue.

The Three Square Meals a Day Myth

Quit counting. Learn to eat when your body is hungry—four, even five times a day. Then wait a couple of hours to give your body a couple of hours to digest, rest, detoxify, and build.

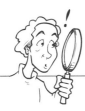

Age Alert

Many time-honored concepts about food—such as a balanced meal must include meat and potatoes—are misconceptions. These ideas must be recognized as myths and dealt with accordingly.

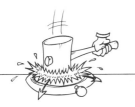

Time Stopper

Did you know that your body requires fat to make the hormones that keep you young? Since hormone production diminishes with age, the inclusion of wisely chosen fats in the diet is essential. These include fresh, raw nuts, avocados, olives and olive oil, flax seed oil, and, yes, coconut.

Keeping your appetite appeased will deter binge eating, because blood-sugar levels, which trigger hunger, will be stabilized.

The Eat Less, Weigh Less Myth

You have to eat to lose weight. It's a myth that fasting or calorie-deprived dieting will make you slim. Also, when you inevitably slip back into your old eating patterns, you'll gain weight back twice as fast.

Long fasts—more than four days at a time—can do more damage than good. Fasting can put your body in famine mode, slowing down the metabolism and overstressing the kidneys and liver. The accumulated toxins that pour into the bloodstream during a fast can cause irreparable damage that may not show up until much later—especially after repeated fasts. Also avoid extremely low-calorie diets.

If you want your body to keep working, you have to keep feeding it the proper fuel.

The Very Low Fat Myth

Fat is necessary to metabolize, or burn, the calories in the food you eat and to satisfy your hunger. Without fat, your metabolism slows down and your energy level drops.

Not getting enough fat in your diet causes premature aging—especially dry, wrinkled skin. The trick is to get your fats from natural sources—nuts, avocados, olives, cold processed oils, etc.—instead of from chemically or heat-extracted fats, hydrogenated cooking oils, or processed foods.

We have been led to believe that a very low-fat diet is the healthiest possible form of eating. So before you become completely caught up in a fat-free frenzy, listen to what the experts have to say. You may be in for a few surprises.

First off, a completely fat-*free* diet is potentially dangerous. The body actually needs fat for optimum health, just as it needs protein and carbohydrates. Fats help to keep the body warm, especially during cold weather. Fats help keep your cell walls strong, and they help you absorb and store fat-soluble vitamins (such as vitamin D, which is needed for the body to absorb calcium from the intestines). Insufficient stores of vitamin D and calcium can lead to bone thinning.

The All Whole Grains Are Great Myth

If you combine even the best organic grains with animal protein, you will slow down your digestive process and clog up your intestines. It's not just the *quality* of the grain, it's what you combine it with that counts.

Also, many whole grains contain a high level of *gluten*. Gluten causes mucous to form and often triggers allergic reactions. Millet, wild rice, and quinoa are lowest in gluten; wheat ranks very high.

The Rice and Beans Myth

It's been proven that you don't have to have *all* of your amino acids at the same meal to have the benefits of a complete protein. As long as you have a balance of nutrients in the course of a day, your body will synthesize the nutrients it needs.

Even though you've heard that rice and beans are a perfect protein meal, we recommend splitting them into two meals. In fact, combining rice and beans in the same meal is difficult to digest and can make you sluggish.

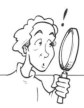

Age Alert

Just slashing the fat from our diets isn't the only way to do damage. When commercial food processors take fat out of a recipe, they have to replace it with something. What they generally choose are gums, sugars, starches, and chemicals. Consequently, the terms "low-fat" and "fat-free" don't mean low-calorie or healthy. In fact, they often indicate that the product is full of nonnutritive, if not downright destructive, ingredients.

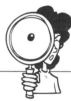

WatchWord

Gluten is the gray, sticky substance found in the flour of wheat and other grains that gives dough its tough, elastic quality. Intolerance to gluten has been implicated in a wide variety of allergies—especially of the digestive system.

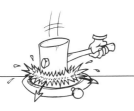

Time Stopper

Dietary fiber helps us stay healthy by preventing constipation, and in certain forms, it helps to lower cholesterol levels and prevent cancer. You'll find fiber in fruits, vegetables, beans, and grains. Soluble fiber—such as that found in oatmeal and oat bran, barley bran, legumes, and dried beans—dissolves in water and is helpful in lowering cholesterol. Insoluble fiber—found in nuts, fruits, and vegetables—is what Grandma called "roughage" and helps prevent constipation and colon cancer.

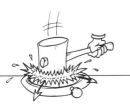

Time Stopper

Cows eat grass and oats to produce milk. No cow alive will drink pasteurized milk. Just remember: Cow's milk is meant for baby cows, which we're not.

A better meal plan:

➤ Beans and greens, leave out the rice, or

➤ Rice and greens, leave out the beans.

Notice how greens are perfect combined with either.

The Sugar for Energy Myth

Refined sugar and snacks containing refined sugar may give you a rapid energy boost, but they will ultimately drop you below where you started. It's like flash powder—poof! You're better off eating complex carbohydrates, which the body slowly turns into sugar that it can use.

Look into unrefined, or raw, sugar, honey, stevia, pure maple syrup, molasses, concentrated fruit, and dried fruit puree as more stable sources of energy. Corn syrup and fructose are to be avoided.

Another component of this myth: Sugar does *not* cause diabetes.

The Carbohydrate Addiction Myth

A healthy body craves carbohydrates for energy; however, not all carbohydrates are equal.

The addiction problem comes when all we eat are refined carbs—white bread, pastries, white rice, etc. What we need are complex carbohydrates from natural, unprocessed sources—whole-grain breads, sprouted grains. These feed the appetite and not the addiction.

The Dairy for Calcium Myth

It is not true that the only way to get calcium is from dairy products. Cows and goats—providers of milk, cheese, butter, etc.—get *their* calcium from the grasses and grains they eat. So the calcium in dairy products is "secondhand."

You'd be smart to go to the source—dark green vegetables like broccoli, kale, chard, and spinach, as well as wheatgrass juice, for example, are high in natural calcium.

Remember: You also need magnesium to process calcium, so make sure that you eat plenty of unsulfured dried fruits.

The Protein Myth—a.k.a. the Everybody Needs Meat Myth

Protein mania has many people—even so-called experts—saying that everybody needs meat. Every nutrient necessary for health and energy can be found in fruits, vegetables, legumes, and grains. And they're in a form that is easily assimilated and digested by the body, with fewer hormones, pesticides, and saturated fats. And, as a bonus, there is no naturally occurring cholesterol in any nonanimal food.

Contrary to popular belief, coconut and coconut oil contain no cholesterol whatsoever.

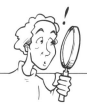

Age Alert

Certain youth-stealing foods are proven binge-starters. Usual ingredients are sugar, salt, and fat. Not surprisingly, most American palates are trained toward these three tastes so we'll eat more. Most commercially produced peanut butters, for example, have both sugar *and* salt in them, and hydrogenated oil to give it the right texture—that smoothness and what the experts call "mouth texture."

The Protein Myth Quiz

True	False	
_____	_____	The human body needs 100 or more grams of protein per day—about 40 grams per meal—for optimum health.
_____	_____	The only way to guarantee that you are eating adequate amounts of protein is to eat fish, poultry, and meat or dairy products every day.
_____	_____	Vegetarians need protein supplements to make sure that they are getting enough protein to build muscles, blood, and new tissue.

If you said *true* to even one of these statements, you have bought into the protein myth.

179

Clearing the Way

Can you hear the sound of all these myths falling? Just like urban renewal, demolition of misinformation is the first step in clearing the path for new growth.

The Least You Need to Know

➤ A food plan must be delicious and satisfying for us to stay with it.

➤ Many foods that you may have thought of as simply unhealthy are in fact hazardous to your health.

➤ The word "nonfoods" applies to anything we eat or drink that is detrimental to our health and ages us prematurely.

➤ The term "youth-foods" refers to anything we eat and drink that nourish us.

➤ Food myths abound and keep us overweight, exhausted, sick, and prematurely old.

Chapter 18

Food-Combining and Other Breakthroughs

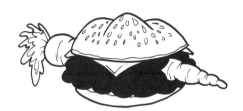

> **In This Chapter**
>
> ➤ Pioneers in the health food movement
>
> ➤ Food-combining—the magic formula
>
> ➤ Super Dense Nutrients—powerful plant-based foods
>
> ➤ Free radicals, antioxidants, and phytonutrients
>
> ➤ Eating for a lifetime of youth
>
> ➤ The trick to eating in restaurants

In case you're worrying that you'll have nothing to eat, now that we've alerted you that so many of the things you've enjoyed eating all your life are nonfoods … relax. There'll be plenty of great youth foods to enjoy.

We'll be teaching you how to eat to satisfaction by combining food in a biologically efficient way. Added to that are what we call *Super Dense Nutrients* (*SDNs*)—delicious, back-to-nature whole foods. Eat this way, and you'll be rewarded with renewed youth and boundless energy as a welcome by-product.

The Origins of the Health Food Movement

Food-combining is not a new idea. The concept has been around since the early 1900s. In those days, it was practiced only by small groups of health-conscious souls who were undoubtedly viewed as fanatics by the meat-and-potatoes-eating public.

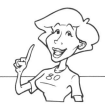

Voice of Experience

For more than 70 years, Dr. Norman W. Walker, D.Sc., was recognized throughout the world as one of the most authoritative students of life, health, and nutrition. In 1910, he began his research of man's ability to live a longer and healthier life. In his 1949 book, *Become Younger* (Norwalk Press), he wrote: "I have found that the correct selection and combination of foods is extremely important if we want to become younger. It is a pitiful and lamentable fact that the vast majority of people simply dig their graves with their teeth and eat themselves into their graves ... in spite of the super abundance of knowledge and proven facts we have today. By studying with an open mind the simple means and methods which nature has made available to every one of us, we can not only defer a premature demise, but actually become younger by putting these into practice."

These hardy individuals formed the nucleus of what has grown to become the health food movement. These were the people who invented graham crackers and shredded-wheat cereals. They even had a song to champion their cause:

Blackstrap molasses and the wheat-germ bread
Make you live so long you'll wish you were dead.
Add some yogurt and you'll be well-fed,
Blackstrap molasses and the wheat-germ bread.

Hattie pulled this ditty from the deep recesses of her memory. She has no idea where she picked it up, but then she also knows the Chinese National Anthem ... in English, no less.

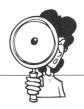

WatchWord

These **Super Dense Nutrients (SDNs)** are natural whole foods rich in essential fatty acids, proteins, enzymes, and minerals that provide your body with all the raw materials necessary for building youth and maintaining a healthy, fit body for a lifetime.

Pioneers in Health

Long before the more well-known proponents of healthy eating (Gayelord Hauser, Dr. Carlton Fredericks, Adele Davis, Dr. William Howard Hay, Dr. John Harvey Kellogg, Paul Bragg, Linda Clark, Bernard Jensen, Marsh Morrison, and John Christopher), there were outspoken practitioners around the world. Among the most notable were George Bernard Shaw, Bernarr Macfadden, and Count Leo Tolstoy.

They were at the vanguard of this health-oriented movement.

Taking a New Look at an Old Idea

More recently, there are Marilyn and Harvey Diamond, whose best-selling book *Fit for Life* popularized the term "food-combining" in the early 1980s. This is the style of eating we endorse for lifelong youth.

The world-renowned motivational guru Anthony Robbins has also recommended food-combining to countless individuals participating in his self-empowerment programs.

Now we'll explain not only how to do it, but why you should.

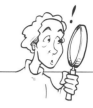

Age Alert

Everyone's heard the adage "You are what you eat." To this we add, "You are what you *don't* eat, too." Unless you eliminate nonfoods, you'll never stay young.

Why Food-Combining?

The way you combine foods impacts your weight, energy, youthfulness, and overall health. Back in the 1930s, William Howard Hay, M.D., was the first to note the strong correlation between wellness and the foods his patients ate.

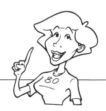

Voice of Experience

More from Dr. Walker: "You have probably eaten an average of three meals a day as a matter of habit. This means you have averaged about a thousand meals a year. If you are 40 years old or more, you have consumed more than 40,000 meals in your lifetime so far. The question for you to ponder now is this: How many of those meals were actually able to furnish the cells and tissues of your body with the real, live, vital nourishment they need for replenishment, reproduction, and regeneration? Look at yourself in your mirror, and you will most likely find the answer written in every line on your face and neck, in every pore of your skin, and in every contour and outline of your body where it sticks out where it shouldn't."

Hattie, who is now a vegetarian, became an advocate of healthy food-combining when she was still eating animal products. "I studied how my own body responded to certain foods and discovered that the only way I could eat to satisfaction and stay healthy was to food-combine. That meant never eating animal proteins—meat and fish, cheese, eggs, milk, yogurt, etc.—and starchy carbohydrates at the same meal. My clients who had weight and digestive problems use this method with great success."

Following Dr. Hay's lead, Hattie categorized foods into two groups:

Group 1: Starchy Complex Carbohydrates

Group 2: Animal Proteins

All Foods Are Not Digested Equally

The starchy complex carbohydrates in Group 1 include starches, grains, and sugars—such as cereals, potatoes, corn, pumpkins, and dry fruits. These carbohydrates begin digesting in the mouth, where ptyalin in the saliva splits them into dextrose (sugars). Then they pass through the acidic stomach to continue the process in the alkaline medium found in the intestines.

The concentrated animal proteins in Group 2—meat, poultry, fish, and seafood, as well as cheese and other dairy products—need the strong digestive fluids, pepsin and hydrochloric acid, found in the stomach to release their nutrients.

The Principles of Food-Combining

Group 1: Starchy Complex Carbohydrates

Wheat, rice, barley, quinoa and other grains, beans and peas, potatoes, winter squashes, corn, breads, pasta, tofu, tempeh, popcorn, chips, pretzels, cereals, raw nuts, seeds, and nut and seed butters.

When you eat starchy complex carbohydrates, eat only vegetables, cooked or raw, including salads, with them. Remember: Absolutely **no animal protein.** It doesn't matter if it's just a splash of grated cheese, sour cream, yogurt, or mayonnaise. It's the chemical composition, not the quantity that counts.

Group 2: Animal Proteins

Beef, chicken, turkey, all fowl, fish (canned and fresh), pork, veal, eggs, milk, cheese, yogurt, and all dairy products.

When you eat animal proteins, you should not have even a mouthful of any form of starch. This includes even a teeny baked potato, a few potato chips, or corn on the cob. **No bread can be eaten with any meal that contains animal protein.**

Never eat foods from Group 1 with foods from Group 2.

You can eat nonstarchy vegetables, like zucchini, broccoli, cauliflower, string beans, eggplant, etc., and green salads with both groups.

184

What Happens When They Combine?

When you eat carbohydrates and proteins in the same meal, your body has a dilemma: It needs a strong alkaline medium for carbohydrate digestion and a strong acid medium for protein digestion.

Remember your high school chemistry: Alkalines and acids neutralize one another. That's what happens when the body is forced to contend with the simultaneous consumption of these two types of food.

When both are in the stomach at the same time, this presents a problem. As Dr. Walker explains: "The digestion of the carbohydrates is interfered with by the presence of the acid material, and at the same time the digestion of the proteins remains incomplete in the presence of the alkaline digestive juices. The result is the fermentation of the carbohydrate and the putrefaction of the protein foods."

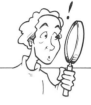

Age Alert

Never have fruit or fruit juices with your meals. You may have them a half hour before or one hour after. Otherwise, you risk digestive troubles: gas, flatulence, discomfort, bloating.

Simple Rules for Food-Combining

Healthy food-combining comes down to a few basic rules:

Rule 1   When you eat proteins, eat them only with nonstarchy vegetables.

Rule 2   Never eat starchy complex carbohydrate foods with animal proteins.

Rule 3   Fruits and fruit juices should *not* be combined with any other food.

Rule 4   Never drink beverages—not even water—with meals, because this dilutes the digestive fluids. The only exception is moderate amounts of wine, preferably red.

Rule 5   Eliminate all nonfoods from both Group 1 and Group 2.

Rule 6   To aid digestion, always include some raw vegetables and/or salad when eating foods from either group to provide essential enzymes not present in cooked foods.

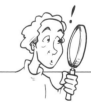

Age Alert

Did you know that there are between 70 and 100 *trillion* cells in your body? And they all need to be fed. If you feed them the nutrients they need, they will stay young, and so will you.

Comfort Foods That Leave You Uncomfortable

Almost all traditional meals—meat and potatoes, turkey and stuffing, spaghetti and meatballs, macaroni and cheese, chicken and rice, fish and chips, and pizza, the "ultimate one-dish meal"—go against the principles of good food-combining. Think of how stuffed and lethargic everyone feels after a big dinner. That's the immediate effect of eating foods in improper combinations. In the long run, this presents serious dangers to your health.

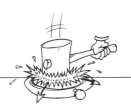

Time Stopper

While we shouldn't drink water with meals, we do need water—and lots of it—for our bodies to be able to function normally. In fact, conditions like heartburn and headaches are early signs of water shortage. Heartburn indicates dehydration in the upper gastrointestinal system, while headaches, especially migraines, signal the brain's need for more water.

A Lifetime of Change

Food-combining is a lifetime change, not just a temporary solution. Weight control, health, and enduring youth depend on your satisfaction, not martyrdom.

The body holds on to old habits, so it may take you time to master this concept. Don't be angry with yourself for occasional backslides or even binges. A healthy body can handle them.

Those SDNs

You'd have to be living under a rock not to have heard words like *free radicals, antioxidants,* and *phytonutrients* bandied about by proponents of healthful eating. A diet based on Super Dense Nutrients provides both antioxidants and phytonutrients in abundance.

While the thrust of the program we recommend is vegetarian, this plan accommodates all eating styles. Food-combining works for everyone as the best means of achieving unprecedented age reversal.

Super Dense Nutrients (SDNs)

Nuts (all unroasted)
Almonds (soaked before use)
   Walnuts
   Macadamias
   Filberts
   Hazelnuts
   Cashews
   Pecans

Super Dense Nutrients (SDNs)

Seeds

    Sunflower

    Flax

    Sesame

    Pumpkin

Nut and seed butters (except for peanut butter)

Soy products and whole grains

    Tofu

Tempeh (high-protein, partially cooked, fermented soybeans)

Soy, almond, and rice milks

Miso (a thick, fermented paste of cooked soybeans, rice or barley, and salt; often used to make soups and sauces)

Sprouted grain cereals and breads

Carrot and root families

    Carrots

    Celery

    Cilantro

    Parsnips

    Beets

    Ginger

Onion family

    Onions

    Garlic

    Scallions

    Shallots

    Leeks

    Chives

Teas

    Green tea

    Herbal teas

Cruciferous vegetables

Broccoli

Cabbage

Brussels sprouts

Cauliflower

Bok choy (Chinese cabbage)

    Radishes

    Daikon (white radish from Japan)

continues

continued

Super Dense Nutrients (SDNs)

Dark green vegetables
> Kale
>
> Spinach
>
> Chard
>
> Turnip and mustard greens
>
> Collards
>
> Watercress
>
> Zucchini
>
> Beet tops

Orange and red vegetables
> Sweet potatoes and yams
>
> Winter and yellow squash
>
> Corn
>
> Tomatoes

Red and yellow peppers
> Hot chiles

Citrus fruits
> Oranges
>
> Red and pink grapefruits
>
> Lemons
>
> Limes
>
> Kiwis

Red, orange, and blue fruits
> Cherries
>
> Bananas
>
> Red grapes
>
> Apples
>
> Strawberries
>
> Raspberries
>
> Watermelons and cantaloupes
>
> Apricots
>
> Blueberries
>
> Plums
>
> Peaches
>
> Papaya

Look at the Whole Week

The American Heart Association has revised its nutritional guidelines to foster flexibility in food selection, suggesting that we consider our food intake *over the course of the week* instead of day by day.

This enables us to consume a *variety* of foods from every food group, sweet, tart, and sour; smooth or crunchy, soft and hard. This is crucial to maintaining a healthy diet.

A Dream Come True

This way of eating frees you of all calorie-counting and portion control. Once you've mastered the principles of food-combining and are consciously consuming SDNs so packed with nutrients they guarantee health and energy, you'll find that your cravings have changed.

What a great feeling to know that destructive food addictions no longer have a hold on you. Because you no longer want them, they won't be throwing your system into a tailspin.

Perhaps you've heard the story of an experiment that tested the food choices of children. When faced with a variety of foods, the test group, without prompting, picked the ones that were best for them.

There was one catch in the original experiment: *All the food offered was healthy.* These children did not have the option of chocolate cake, candy bars, or ice cream sundaes. We suspect that had they been available, the children might have chosen them, just as we do. And just like us, once they've chosen the "goody," the "good" loses its appeal.

Have you ever experienced going on a diet and suddenly realizing how delicious radishes, carrots, tomatoes, and celery taste? Then, of course, as soon as you have one serving of a rich food or dessert, your palate loses its delight in the pure foods. You start craving and eating foods that are complicated, with sugars, sauces, gravies, seasonings, and multiple ingredients.

WatchWord

Free radicals are unstable molecules with unpaired electrons in their outer shell. They seek to steal an electron from another molecule and often destroy healthy cells in the process. One of the best ways to combat free-radical damage is to consume plenty of **antioxidants.** This includes foods and supplements that are high in vitamins C and E and beta-carotene. Antioxidants also keep the formation of new free radicals in check.

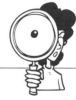

WatchWord

Phytonutrients are intensely rich nutritional elements with outstanding healing properties. They are found only in edible plants.

189

To eat healthily, you must keep cleaning up your food intake and adding copious amounts of SDNs.

Rules in Restaurants

If restaurants throw you into such a dietary spin that you say *fugeddaboutit* the minute you open the menu, here are some ways to make sure you stick to your food plan—wherever and whenever you dine:

➤ Before you order, decide if you're going to have a meal with protein in it. In that way, you can ask the waiter to substitute a salad or green vegetable for the usual starchy side dishes like potatoes, rice, or pasta.

➤ Request that the waiter not serve you water. The *only* permissible beverage during meals is wine in moderation. No exceptions.

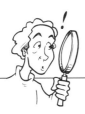

Age Alert

The more processed and complicated your food intake, the more you will crave unhealthy, fattening, youth-stealing foods.

➤ Don't let the waiter leave that tempting basket of white rolls and breadsticks for you to mindlessly munch on while waiting for your meal. Request a bowl of crudités instead.

➤ Even if the bread is made of nutritious whole grains, you can't eat it if you plan to have any animal protein at your meal.

➤ And, sorry to say, skip dessert, coffee, and brandy. Even fresh fruit, however healthy, isn't good for you after a meal. Wait at least an hour.

➤ And, in case you're tempted to reward yourself for good behavior, skip the free mints at the cash register.

The Least You Need to Know

➤ The health food movement has been quietly growing for more than a century.

➤ Food-combining means never eating complex carbohydrates and proteins in the same meal.

➤ A diet of Super Dense Nutrients (SDNs) is essential to combat disease and ensure rejuvenation.

➤ Be careful when dining out. Restaurants are infamous for pulling you off-track.

190

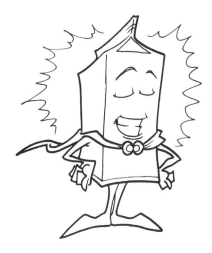

Food, Glorious Food!

Now that we've told you that you'll have to make some serious changes in how and what you eat if you're going to grow younger, it's time to tell you how to implement them.

You'll start by Blitzing all nonfoods from your kitchen. Then you'll shop with far greater awareness, stocking your larder with super-healthy and super-delicious youth foods that you can enjoy without guilt.

This chapter is controversial because we recommend switching to a plant-based diet. The evidence keeps building that vegetarianism is the most powerful youth- and health-providing mode of eating.

We acknowledge that this won't be everyone's choice. Nevertheless, we are convinced that following a vegetarian diet will make you look and feel younger starting now.

There's also the issue of killing animals to satisfy our appetites. Our favorite vegan restaurant, the Candle Café in New York City, sports a sticker on the front door: "Be kind to animals. Don't eat them."

Let's Blitz Again

Grab a jumbo box of heavy-duty trash bags and get ready to fill them. You're in for a big surprise at how many things you've kept in your cupboards long past their expiration dates—like the box of oatmeal to be used before April 1992 Sallie found when moving from a summer house in 1998. Granted, wine may improve with age, but oatmeal?

You'll certainly find examples of your own, just as you'll be amazed at the mountain of nonfoods you once considered staples—canned corned beef, spaghetti and meatballs, fruit cocktail in heavy syrup, etc.—and saved in case of a power failure. You probably bought most of these on sale. Three cans for a dollar is no deal if what's in them is damaging to your health!

Beginning Your Blitz

You may want to set aside an entire day to Blitz your kitchen. Or, if you think the sight of so many groceries going out the door all at once might overwhelm you, spread it out over a few days.

The only caveat is that you not run to the supermarket to immediately restock your almost empty shelves. Wait until you have completed your Blitz. Then make a thorough shopping list of youth foods to replace the nonfoods you've discarded.

Kitchen Blitz Checklist

We divide this Blitz process into three categories: throwaways, possible keepers (which we call *transitionals*), and keepers.

➤ **Throwaways.** You once called them foods, but now that you know they're nonfoods, get rid of them. These include refined flours and sugars; anything with most preservatives—nitrates in particular; and artificial sweeteners, flavors, and coloring.

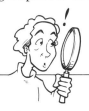

Age Alert

When Blitzing your home of all unhealthy foods (nonfoods), get them out immediately. Experience has shown that if they're still around, they'll end up back on the shelves—or in your mouth.

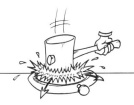

Time Stopper

Don't feel anxious at the sight of an empty fridge and bare cupboards. Your kitchen won't stay empty long. After Blitzing all nonfoods, you'll have plenty of room to restock your shelves for a whole new way of eating for youth. Congratulate yourself for your courage. Clearing the way for change isn't easy.

Refrigerator/Freezer

Ice cream

Frozen yogurt

Frozen microwaveable meals

Sodas and juice drinks

Whole-milk products

Bottled salad dressings, mayonnaise, and ketchup (high in refined sugar)

Canola oil

Processed meats (all contain carcinogenic nitrates)

Anything fried

Pantry/Cupboards

White flour, white pasta, macaroni products

White rice

Cake mixes

Prepackaged pastries

Fried chips, canned chili, canned ham

Canned almost anything

Gelatin and pudding mixes

➤ **Transitionals.** Foods that you may not be ready to give up are possible keepers. We like to think of them as *transitionals*—foods that aren't healthy but are not toxic. If you're working toward becoming a vegetarian, add meat, fowl, fish, and dairy products to this list of transitionals.

Refrigerator/Freezer

Sorbets and frozen juice pops

Commercial peanut butter (with sugar, salt, and hydrogenated oil)

Nonsweetened juice concentrates

Bottled salsa and relishes

Pickles

Low fat milk

Cheese

Chicken

Eggs

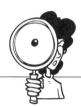

WatchWord

On the path of refining how we eat, there are still some items that are difficult to eliminate. Ultimately, we will eliminate these **transitionals,** even though we may not be quite ready to do it all at once.

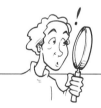

Age Alert

If there's only one food that you must choose to be organic, let it be eggs. Commercial eggs are potentially dangerous. Not only are the chickens that lay them treated abominably, their eggs are laden with hormones, antibiotics, and pesticides. Avoid them at all costs.

Pantry/Cupboards

Marmalades, jellies, and jams

Canned tuna and salmon

Juice-packed fruits

Popcorn

Coffee

Honey-roasted nuts

➤ **Keepers.** The first time you Blitz your food supply, you may not have many keepers—unless you're already in the habit of eating fresh fruits and vegetables and whole-grain products.

Refrigerator/Freezer	**Pantry/Cupboards**
Soy- and rice-milk ice creams	Whole-grain crackers
All fresh or flash-frozen fruits and vegetables, preferably organic	Rice cakes, whole-grain pastas, brown rice
Whole- or sprouted-grain breads, all nuts and seeds	Dried spices and herbs
Unsulfured dried fruits	Herbal teas
Roasted sesame oil	Green tea
Extra-virgin olive oil	
Coconut oil	
Whole-grain flours	
Steel-cut oatmeal	
Soy, almond, and rice milk	
Pickles and sauerkraut without vinegar	

The Truth About Protein

Contrary to what you learned in fifth-grade health class, we do *not* need massive quantities of protein to build a healthy body. Instead of 40 to 50 grams per *meal*, our bodies require a mere 40 to 50 grams per *day*.

Beef/pork/poultry/seafood/dairy producers may want us to believe protein only comes from the animal kingdom, but that's not true. Grains, legumes, green leafy vegetables, and nuts and seeds are absolutely power-packed with protein without cholesterol.

Building Blocks for Youth

While protein is a necessary nutrient, providing the body with the building blocks that make muscles, blood, hormones, and new tissue (including hair, fingernails, and skin), research shows that most Americans consume as much as five times more protein than is needed to meet their actual metabolic needs.

The truth is, the traditional American meat-and-potatoes diet is not good for your health, not to mention that it also violates the principles of food-combining.

The protein found in animal muscle tissue is far more concentrated than the plant protein found in whole grains, dark green vegetables, and legumes, consequently overloading the body with each meat-laden meal. A meat meal acts much like an electrical power surge, zapping the system with enough protein to cause potential damage to the kidneys and liver. Clogging the renal filters can lead to kidney failure and liver damage.

Concentrated animal protein has also been proven to leach calcium from the bones, leading to osteoporosis. In contrast, a balanced vegetarian diet supplies the body's protein needs without dealing a damaging blow.

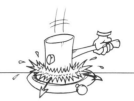

Time Stopper

Think of a Blitz as throwing out your mistakes, and stop worrying about the money you spent on these foods. You didn't know they weren't good for you when you bought them, so don't blame yourself. In this case, worrying about money is definitely penny-wise and *age*-foolish.

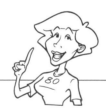

Voice of Experience

Dr. Michael Klaper, an outspoken advocate of meatless nutrition, states "The idea of plant protein being incomplete and lacking some amino acids has been shown to be a myth. Nature simply cannot make a soybean, potato, or grain of wheat without using all the same amino acids (the building blocks of protein) required by the metabolism of humans."

The Four Potent Veggie Protein Groups

If you eat from these four groups of foods, you'll get all the complete protein you need:

Group 1:   Whole grains—millet, corn, barley, brown rice, wild rice, kasha, quinoa, amaranth, etc.

Group 2:   Legumes—lentils, chick peas, alfalfa sprouts, and beans of all kinds—adzuki, lima, soy, and products made from them.

195

Group 3:   Dark green vegetables—kale, collard greens, broccoli, spinach, broccoli raab, beet tops, etc.

Group 4:   Nuts and seeds—almonds, cashews, walnuts, pecans, pistachios, macadamias, and nut butters made from them, with the exception of peanut butter.

Fill Up with Fiber

One of the most important food components you eat has no nutrient value whatsoever: fiber. Plant foods are replete with it. Animal muscle has next to no fiber, which is why people who eat lots of meat have a high incidence of colon cancer.

There are two types of fiber:

➤ **Soluble fiber.** Found in oatmeal and oat bran, barley bran, legumes, and dried beans. Dissolves in water and is helpful in lowering cholesterol.

➤ **Insoluble fiber.** Found in wheat and corn bread, nuts, fruits, and vegetables. What grandma called "roughage" helps prevent constipation and colon cancer.

For a lifetime of youth and health, eat a variety of fruit, vegetables, grains, and legumes so that you get sufficient soluble and insoluble fiber.

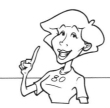

Voice of Experience

Says Hattie: "We've been warned to avoid oily foods, lest we get fat. What actually happens when we do that is that we starve our organs and cells. Every single day, I eat an abundance of unprocessed foods that naturally contain a high fat content, yes, even organic chocolate, and I never put on an ounce. My clients were afraid of putting on weight if they ate avocados, olives, nuts. They didn't—and you won't either."

Facts About Fats

Food contains three basic types of fat: saturated, polyunsaturated, and monounsaturated.

➤ Not all saturated fats are alike. There are two groups—medium and long chain—and each acts differently in the body.

Long-chain saturates are found primarily in animal products like fat from meat, butter, cheese, and other milk products. These pose a serious danger to the body, most significantly by boosting levels of "bad" cholesterol (LDL) and lowering levels of "good" cholesterol (HDL). They also contribute to certain cancers, especially colon and prostate. These must be eliminated from the diet.

Medium-chain saturates from plant sources such as coconuts are easily digested and do not clog arteries. Because coconut oil is naturally saturated, it never needs to be hydrogenated—the process that changes fat from liquid to solid at room temperature. This turns the fatty acids into harmful trans fatty acids (TFAs).

➤ Polyunsaturated fats are primarily vegetable oils, such as corn and soy oil, and products made from liquid vegetable oils, such as homemade salad dressings—tend to lower cholesterol levels, yet when heated they have been found to be easily susceptible to the dangers of free-radical chemical reactions which accelerate aging.

Processed polyunsaturated fats—commercially prepared salad dressings, hydrogenated margarines and toppings such as butter substitutes used on popcorn—should also be eliminated. Unprocessed, cold-pressed polyunsaturated oils can be used safely, but never in cooking because they break down when heated forming free radicals.

➤ Monounsaturated fats—found in olives, avocados, and nuts, mainly hazelnuts and almonds—help lower damaging LDL cholesterol levels. They contain antioxidants that combat clogging of the arteries and chronic diseases, including cancer. These are healthy and should be eaten daily.

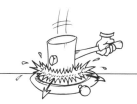

Time Stopper

Coconut oil has been given a bum rap. Almost 50 percent of the fatty acids in cold-pressed coconut oil is lauric acid, a disease-fighting fatty acid. This makes it ideal for immune-suppressed individuals. Lauric acid is also found naturally in mother's milk, protecting infants from viral and bacterial infections.

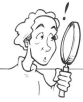

Age Alert

Originally known as "rapeseed oil," canola oil is being challenged as a safe and suitable food source. According to Essential Oils Online, this semi-drying plant oil that is also used as a lubricant, fuel, and synthetic rubber base, has been linked to Mad Cow disease in animals and Alzheimer's disease in humans. It was banned in Europe in 1991. To date, it is still used as a commercial food additive in the United States. Read labels carefully and avoid its use.

There Are Fats, and Then There Are Fats

Since not all fats are created equal, it's helpful to know which *kinds* of fats you are consuming. The catch is that not all fats are good for us.

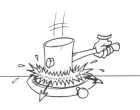

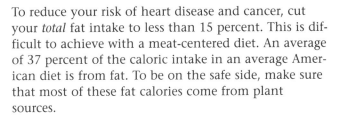

To reduce your risk of heart disease and cancer, cut your *total* fat intake to less than 15 percent. This is difficult to achieve with a meat-centered diet. An average of 37 percent of the caloric intake in an average American diet is from fat. To be on the safe side, make sure that most of these fat calories come from plant sources.

Fatty Acids Pack a Wallop

In the "healthy fat" category you will also find EFAs—Essential Fatty Acids. They are getting quite a bit of attention because they function as building blocks in the membranes of every cell in the body. They also produce hormone-like *prostoglandins* that are necessary for energy metabolism and cardiovascular and immune health.

Fatty acids are the major components of all fats. To maintain normal function, the body uses 20 specific fatty acids. All but two can be synthesized by the body. The two that must be obtained from foods or supplements are Omega 3 and Omega 6. While both are found in fish liver oils, unrefined flax seed oil is an outstanding source of this polyunsaturated oil. This oil must never be used for cooking. It must be refrigerated. Take one to three tablespoons daily.

Recipe Makeovers

Even though you're committed to changing your diet to support your quest to look and feel younger, you'll still want to eat some of the dishes you've always loved.

That's not nearly as impossible as it may seem. Here are ways to make smarter choices in the ingredients and cooking methods you use:

➤ Substitute *texturized vegetable protein* (TVP) or *tempeh,* a fermented soy product, for meat in

---

Time Stopper

If you can't completely eliminate cholesterol-laden meat and dairy products from your diet, start by eating one vegetarian meal a day. Then designate an entire meatless *day* a week. Keep adding veggie days to your plan until you eliminate meat and meat foods from your diet altogether. If you slip occasionally, you've still made great progress. Congratulate yourself. Giving up animal products may make you feel deprived in the short run. In the long run, it makes you feel great, physically and ethically.

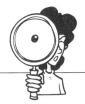

WatchWord

Prostoglandins are hormone-like substances that the body requires for energy metabolism. They also assist in cardiovascular and immune system health.

sauces, stews, and stir-fries. These products are widely available from health food stores and can be found in some supermarkets.

➤ To remove fat from food, especially soups and stews, chill until the fat coagulates on the top and skim it off. Reheat and serve.

➤ Substitute extra-virgin olive oil or coconut oil for hydrogenated solid shortening, including margarine and butter.

➤ Use pureed vegetables, especially starchy root vegetables like carrots, parsnips, turnips, and potatoes, instead of flour to thicken soups and sauces. Remember: Traditional sauces and gravies are hidden sources of fat.

➤ In baking, substitute pureed prunes (or baby-food prunes) for butter or other shortening. The ratio is one-half cup of prunes to replace one cup of butter, margarine, or shortening. You may have to adjust, or possibly eliminate, the amount of sugar in your recipe. If you don't like prunes, experiment with applesauce and mashed bananas.

➤ Add flavor to extra-virgin olive oil or roasted sesame oil by infusing the oil with fresh or dried herbs. Make this fresh every time you use it. Let herbs soak in oil for several hours for the flavors to blend.

➤ If you want to sauté foods, mix a little water with a bit of cold-pressed extra-virgin olive oil or coconut oil. No matter how you've been warned to the contrary, unrefined, nonhydrogenated coconut oil is **not** high in trans fatty acids, and it's stable at high temperatures. As the water evaporates, you'll have that nice "crispy sautéed taste" with very little fat. The only downside: The oil and water spatter a bit. Keep a cover on until the spattering stops.

Sweet Substitutes for Refined Sugars

While maple syrup, raw brown sugar, honey, and molasses are often used as sugar substitutes, they are not without faults. They may contain more vitamins and minerals, but they raise blood-sugar levels every bit as quickly as refined white sugar.

The tasty news is that several safe and natural sweeteners are available. Because they are slow to elevate blood sugar, the body needs to produce very little insulin to control glucose levels. Among these are *stevia,* which is extracted from the Stevia *rebaudiana* plant; *agave,* from the cactus; and KiSweet™, which is made from kiwi fruit. Not yet popularly known, these products may be difficult to find. However, the search is worth the effort. Request that your market stock them for you.

Age Alert

The average American eats approximately 160 pounds of refined sugar a year. Don't be one of them.

199

Fructose is the sugar found naturally in fruit and fruit juices. Often it is used commercially as a substitute for refined sugar. When reading labels, however, make sure that you see "fruit" or "fruit juice," not "fructose" or "fructose syrup." The latter two sweeteners, like corn syrup, have been refined so that they're virtually the same as table sugar.

Read Labels for Youth

If we only ate fresh foods made from scratch, we wouldn't be faced with translating what's written on the labels. Read carefully, and you'll learn more than the calories, kinds of fat, fat and carbohydrate grams, amounts of sodium and sugar (measured in milligrams), and portion size. Here are some things to keep in mind:

➤ When you see the words "low-calorie" on a label, the product can contain no more than 40 calories per serving or per 100 grams (3.5 ounces). The label must substantiate this.

➤ "Reduced-calorie" applies to foods with less than one-third fewer calories than nutritionally comparable foods that are not calorie reduced.

➤ "Dietetic" does not necessarily mean low-calorie. That term can be used to indicate anything intended for special food plans, such as sodium-restricted or reduced-sugar diets.

➤ "Sugar-free" applies to food using artificial sweeteners.

➤ "No sugar added" means that no refined sugars, including high-fructose and corn syrups, are added. This does not exclude use of fruit purees and juices.

➤ "Sodium-free" indicates that the product contains less than five milligrams of sodium per serving.

➤ "Very low sodium" contains 35 milligrams or less of sodium per serving.

➤ "Reduced sodium" means that the food has 75 percent less sodium than comparable foods that do not have reduced sodium.

➤ "Light," "lite," "leaner," or "lower" fat foods must contain 25 percent less fat than comparable, nutritionally equivalent foods.

➤ "Lean" and "low-fat" goods must, by law, contain less than 10 percent fat. "Extra lean" means that a food contains no more than 5 percent fat.

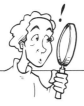

Age Alert

The only essential nutrient not provided in sufficient quantity by a vegetarian diet is vitamin B_{12}, which assists in building red blood cells. It should be taken as a supplement, or a serious form of anemia can result.

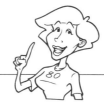

Voice of Experience

Hattie offers this recipe she calls Tempeh Toss as a great introduction to high-protein vegetarian eating. Tempeh, made from fermented soybeans, is easily digested. High in protein (more than 22 grams per four-ounce serving), it takes on the flavors of any herbs, spices, and sauces you add to it. Unlike tofu, which falls apart in cooking, tempeh holds its shape and, for that reason, can be used in much the same way as meat.

Tempeh Toss

2 tablespoons coconut or extra-virgin olive oil
1 small onion, coarsely chopped
1 tablespoon minced raw ginger
One 8-ounce package organic tempeh, cubed
$^1/_8$ cup Bragg's Aminos
Finely chopped parsley to garnish

In a sauté pan, add oil and warm over medium heat. Sauté onions in oil until transparent and lightly browned. Add ginger and tempeh cubes; stir to mix. Continue cooking over medium heat three to four minutes, until warm. Add Bragg's Aminos and bring to a boil while stirring. Garnish with parsley. *Serves two as entrée; four as appetizer.*

Going Veggie

Vegetarians are individuals who base their diets primarily on fruits and vegetables, grains, legumes, seeds, and nuts. Within vegetarianism, there are several varieties, distinguished by the degree to which the individual has eliminated animal products from his or her diet—and, in the case of vegans, from his or her entire life. Here's a rundown:

➤ *Ovo-lacto-vegetarians* consume milk, milk products, and eggs. This diet eliminates all products that involve the killing of animals. Most of the food eaten is from plant sources—fruits, vegetables, legumes, grains, nuts, and seeds.

➤ *Lacto-vegetarians* eat milk and milk products but consume no eggs or other animal products. They follow a predominantly plant-based diet.

201

➤ *Ovo-vegetarians* eat eggs but consume no products from animals that are killed or tortured. Once again, the bulk of this diet consists of plant-based foods.

➤ *Pollo-vegetarians* eat no red meats, but they do eat moderate amounts chicken, eggs, and dairy products in conjunction with a primarily plant-based diet.

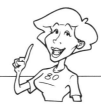

Voice of Experience

The average age (longevity) of a meat eater is 63. I am on the verge of 85 and still work as hard as ever. I have lived quite long enough and am trying to die; but I simply cannot do it. A single beef-steak would finish me; but I cannot bring myself to swallow it. I am oppressed with the dread of living forever. This is the only disadvantage of vegetarianism.

—George Bernard Shaw (1856–1950)

➤ *Pesca-vegetarians* eat no meat or fowl but include some fish, eggs, and dairy products in their plant-based diet.

➤ *Vegans* eat absolutely no products derived from animals—including honey and gelatin (even vitamin capsules, unless vegetable gelatin is used). They avoid wearing leather, wool, or silk, or using any product derived from animals for any reason. Their diet consists solely of plant foods—vegetables, fruits, nuts, seeds, grains, and legumes.

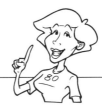

Voice of Experience

I have from an early age abjured the use of meat, and the time will come when men such as I will look upon the murder of animals as they now look upon the murder of men.

—Leonardo da Vinci (1452–1519)

The Least You Need to Know

➤ A kitchen Blitz rids your home of all nonfoods and prepares you for a lifetime of eating for youth.

➤ Vegetables provide more than adequate protein for all your body's needs.

➤ A diet rich in super-dense nutrients keeps you healthy, youthful, and energetic.

➤ The body needs some fat, especially Omega 3 and Omega 6, each day to support metabolism.

➤ Changing ingredients and cooking methods transforms moderately nutritious foods into healthy ones.

➤ A vegetarian diet is insurance against disease and premature aging.

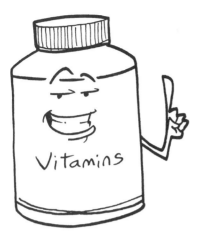

Supplementally Speaking

Vitamins, minerals, herbs … they're everywhere. Once found exclusively in health food stores, they now rival beauty products for shelf space in drug and grocery stores. An increasing number of chain stores and Web sites are dedicated to the sale of these supplements.

It's dizzying.

So what's a body to do? With new products offering astounding claims of health, beauty, and age-reversal emerging almost daily, health seekers are left in a quandary.

Nutrients Once Came Naturally

Once upon a time, before the earth's soil was depleted of microorganisms and other vital nutrients, and our food supply was tainted, everything we needed to stay strong and healthy could be provided by the food we ate. The soil was alive with vast colonies of microorganisms that inhibited disease and rich in minerals and trace elements.

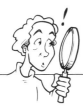

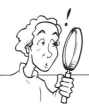

Food grown in this nature-blessed soil provided every possible nutrient to ensure a healthy life. This early soil was richly endowed with the minerals necessary for metabolism: sodium, potassium, calcium, phosphorus, and magnesium—and more than 70 trace elements that the body needs to maintain health.

We're familiar with many of them: iron, iodine, zinc, chromium, copper. But what about holmium, francium, selenium, lithium, thorium, gadolinium, and a bunch more "-iums"? We may not know what they are, but our bodies need tiny amounts of them to function.

Sadly, we can no longer get them from their natural source. Our food cannot get these nutrients from the soil in which it grows; consequently it can't pass them along to us. The amount of fertile topsoil itself has diminished, and what is left is severely nutritiously depleted—and poisoned to boot.

Turning to Supplements for Health

Because we can no longer rely on the food we eat to supply many of the vitamins and minerals essential to life, we must turn to supplements.

If you go into a health food store, you may get the impression that you need to take hundreds of pills a day. Not true. The body is able to synthesize much of what it needs when given the basic raw materials.

Judicious combining of food and supplements will meet your body's needs.

Eleven Vitamins Everybody Needs for Youth

A high-potency natural multivitamin is a good place to start, provided of course that you aren't taking a couple of pills to substitute eating an SDN-rich diet. A good multivitamin contains the following:

➤ **Vitamin A (retinol).** Needed for night vision, bone development, reproduction, and mucus-membrane health. It purifies the blood of toxins that damage new cellular growth. For more youth-producing benefits, choose beta-carotene over the oil-based form of this vitamin.

➤ **B1 (thiamin).** Needed for carbohydrate metabolism and brain, nerve, and muscle functions.

➤ **B2 (riboflavin).** Needed for metabolizing food for energy.

➤ **Niacin.** Needed for metabolizing food for energy. It also boosts the immune system, keeps the skin healthy, and lowers both cholesterol and triglycerides. Do not take timed-release capsules or tablets.

➤ **B6 (pyridoxine).** Helps the body use protein for cell rejuvenation; boosts the immune system and protects cells against cancer.

➤ **B12 (cobalamin).** Helps produce red blood cells. Since this is found only in animal products, vegetarians must take this supplement daily to avoid developing anemia.

➤ **Folacin (folic acid).** Essential for red blood cell production and rebuilding body cells.

➤ **Vitamin C (ascorbic acid).** One of the most powerful age-reversing vitamins, this is necessary for general growth of body cells and also for fighting infection and reducing stress. This is the one vitamin the body is incapable of synthesizing. Though present in food, particularly citrus fruits, the amount is negligible, considering the body's needs. Do not take timed-release capsules or tablets. Look for words like "rose hips," "bioflavonoids," "rutin," and "hespidrin" for natural forms of vitamin C.

➤ **Vitamin D (calciferol).** Essential for the development of bones and teeth. The skin manufactures this when exposed to sunlight. During the winter, or if you spend long periods without being in the sun, this is a necessary supplement.

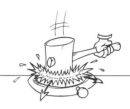

Time Stopper

Make sure your diet is high in folate, also known as folic acid, to combat wintertime weariness. Our bodies use this B-complex nutrient to produce normal red blood cells, to promote wound healing and resist infection, and to synthesize DNA and metabolize protein. This potent infection fighter, found in lentils and other dried beans, can be helpful in combating winter's health woes.

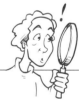

Age Alert

Take all vitamin and mineral supplements with or immediately after meals in order to use the digestive fluids that have been stimulated by eating. Taken on an empty stomach, supplements can cause nausea. At bedtime, they can keep you awake.

207

➤ **Vitamin E (tocopherol).** A powerful antioxidant, this improves circulation, protects cells from degeneration, and aids in new cell growth. It's especially good for your heart, skin, and hair, as well as for cystic mastitis.

➤ **Vitamin K.** Essential for the proper clotting of blood.

Mining for Marvelous Minerals

Minerals are crucial for a variety of body functions, including bone development, red blood cell production, nerve and muscle health, and energy production. Though the amounts needed are much smaller than for vitamins, they are of equal importance to our health.

➤ **Calcium.** Essential for bone and tooth development, blood clotting, and proper muscle function. Calcium is particularly important for postmenopausal women to prevent bone loss.

➤ **Chromium.** Aiding in efficient carbohydrate metabolism, this balances blood-sugar levels and also reduces sugar cravings. It is valuable for individuals on weight-loss programs.

➤ **Copper.** Needed for hemoglobin and red blood cell growth; it also helps prevent bone loss.

➤ **Iodine.** Supports the thyroid gland and assists in hormone production.

➤ **Iron.** Essential for hemoglobin; oxygenates tissues for energy output.

➤ **Magnesium.** Supports the function of nerves, the storage and release of energy, and muscle contraction, particularly of the heart. Magnesium, taken at bedtime, often relieves muscle spasms, especially in the legs.

➤ **Manganese.** Fosters bone health. A powerful antioxidant, it plays a strong role in cellular regeneration.

➤ **Methyl Sulfunyl Methane (MSM).** This essential mineral is present in every cell of the body, with the highest concentration in the joints, hair, skin, and nails; helpful in alleviating arthritis.

➤ **Molybdenum.** This strong antioxidant detoxifies the body of poisons from the air, food, and water that invade the body daily.

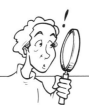

Age Alert

We cannot stress it strongly enough: Choose vitamins only from food sources—organic whenever possible. Although synthetic vitamins have the necessary components, they are produced artificially. The body has more than enough chemicals to contend with. Buy from companies with long, established reputations and expect to pay more for their experience and quality controls.

➤ **Potassium.** Necessary for nerve function and muscle activity; good for the heart.

➤ **Phosphorus.** Needed for bone strength and energy.

➤ **Selenium.** Protects cells from damage. This antioxidant boosts the immune system and protects the heart, liver, and pancreas.

➤ **Sodium.** Maintains body-fluid balance. While the body may be deficient in other minerals, it generally has more than enough sodium.

➤ **Zinc.** Vital for immune-system strength. Helps combat infections, particularly of the throat. Promotes healthy skin and wound healing. It is essential for DNA and RNA production.

Give Us the Edge

Vitamins and minerals have received a great deal of attention in age-reversal. While they are certainly important, they can't do the job on their own.

What's the missing element? *Enzymes.*

Vitamins, minerals, and even food require enzymes in order to be properly assimilated into the system. Otherwise, even these healthy components put stress on the body. Long known as catalysts to all chemical reactions in the body (especially when related to digestion), enzymes have only recently been getting the attention they deserve as being indispensable to life.

To say that we would die without enzymes is not an exaggeration.

How Enzymes Work

Three categories of enzymes affect the body's health:

➤ **Digestive, or intrinsic, enzymes.** These are secreted throughout the digestive system. They break down the food so that the body can use it.

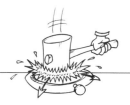

Time Stopper

Selenium has been getting a lot of attention as an antioxidant. It increases the production of enzymes that stop the dangerous oxidation of fats and the production of **low-density lipoprotein** (**LDL**)—the bad cholesterol. Selenium occurs naturally in wheat. Together with vitamin E, it strengthens the immune system and the thyroid function, and keeps the heart, liver, and pancreas healthy. Added to zinc, it can reduce an enlarged prostate.

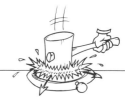

Time Stopper

You'll notice that we haven't told you how much of these vitamins and minerals you should be taking. We believe that each individual has such different requirements that to recommend a specific dosage would be counterproductive. The more abundantly you provide your body with organic SDNs, the fewer supplements you will require. Learn to listen to your body. It will lead you to what it needs.

➤ **Extrinsic digestive enzymes, or food enzymes.** These are found in all raw and fresh food. Unfortunately, the enzymatic activity of this food is diminished, if not completely destroyed, by cooking, preservation, and storage.

➤ **Metabolic enzymes.** These are present in every cell, tissue, and organ, are vital to all bodily functions, including the production of new enzymes, recycling, detoxification, immune-system function, sexual activity, and reproduction. It's impossible to look and feel younger without an ample supply of metabolic enzymes.

Extending the Limits

The catch is that the body's potential to produce enzymes, which is provided at birth, is a limited resource. When the enzyme potential is exhausted beyond a certain point, it triggers the end of the life span.

It's been proven that metabolic enzyme activity drops with aging. For example, *ptyalin,* the enzyme in the saliva, is 30 times stronger in the mouths of young adults than of people past 69. If that's not enough, *amylase,* an enzyme that converts starch to sugar, in urine specimens of young adults is 25; in older people, it's 14.

The good news is that you can augment the body's enzyme supply with supplements, thereby extending your potential life span and fostering youth.

Every Meal, Not Just Every Day

Vitamin and mineral supplements can be taken once a day, or even not at all, especially if you're eating well and drinking freshly squeezed juices. This is not the case with enzymes.

We would be remiss if we didn't strongly urge you to include enzyme supplementation in your program to look and feel younger.

Some 230,000 cells are created each second. That's about 20 billion a day. Each cellular transformation requires thousands of biochemical steps that cannot be complete without metabolic enzymes.

Unfortunately, eating cooked food in tandem with bad eating habits exhausts the body's enzymatic potential.

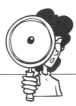

WatchWord

Enzymes are metabolic protein molecules that catalyze or accelerate every biochemical reaction in the body. There *is* no life without enzymes.

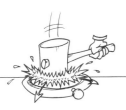

Time Stopper

CoQ_{10}—coenzyme$_{10}$—has been making headlines as a powerful anti-aging compound. Taken as a supplement, it helps activate the body's enzyme system. As an antioxidant, immune system booster, muscle strengthener, and energy producer, it improves physical endurance and is valuable in any youth-enhancing program.

210

With each meal that is enzyme deficient, the body's capacity to regenerate and protect itself diminishes. That's why enzymes must be taken with every meal.

Shopping for Enzymes

Here are the ingredients to look for when you begin shopping for your plant-based enzyme supplements:

➤ **Protein digestion.** *Protease,* which breaks proteins down into peptides. *Peptidase,* which breaks down the peptides into amino acids.

➤ **Carbohydrate digestion.** Amylase, invertase, and maltase and alpha glactosidase, all of which prevent flatulence and bloating.

➤ **Dairy product digestion.** Lactase. People who have low levels of lactase can be lactose intolerant. Lactase can restore digestive balance without the use of antacids.

➤ **Cellulose digestion.** Cellulase. This is essential for the digestion of cellulose—the primary fiber in fruits and vegetables. It's especially important for anyone who eats a high-fiber diet.

➤ **Fat digestion.** Lipase. People who have low levels of lipase are more likely to have elevated LDL cholesterol.

Take supplementary enzymes with every meal, without fail. This will radically transform your aging process by making valuable nutrients available for cellular repair and regeneration.

Choose a product, such as green papaya tablets, capable of digesting both alkaline and acidic foods.

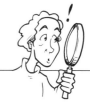

Age Alert

Enzyme supplements must come from a plant source. Animal-sourced or chemically synthesized enzymes are often called *pancreatic enzymes* and are usually indicated by the symbol "USP." These are capable only of digesting protein and not the full range of food groups. Avoid them.

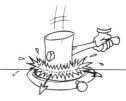

Time Stopper

Scientists at the University of Massachusetts Medical Center have confirmed that the typically low level of protease found in older people reduces their ability to digest and absorb the proteins needed to maintain energy and muscle tone.

Antioxidants: The Body's Youth-Builders

Antioxidants function as powerful free-radical scavengers and fight premature aging and disease. *The Prescription for Nutritional Healing,* by James F. Balch, M.D., and

Phyllis A. Balch, C.N.C. (Avery Publications, 1997), lists 16 references to *superoxide dismutase* (*SOD*) as an aid to fight a weakened immune system, Parkinson's disease, Alzheimer's disease, cardiovascular disease, memory loss, prostate cancer, gout, and other conditions.

In addition to the more popular vitamin C, vitamin E, and beta-carotene, seek out supplements that contain four highly protective enzymes: superoxide dismutase (SOD), *catalase* (*CAT*), glutathione peroxidase, and methionine reductase.

Bonus points: These four protective enzymes guard against wrinkles and age spots.

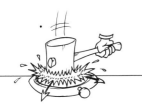

Time Stopper

Raw fruits and vegetables—in particular, freshly squeezed juices—give the body's enzyme levels a major boost. The more fresh juice you drink every day, the healthier and younger you will become. Start juicing!

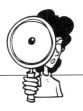

WatchWord

Probiotics are colonies of microorganisms present in the intestines that combat unhealthy bacterial growth. These friendly bacteria are considered a second immune system.

Friendly Bacteria

In the days before penicillin and other antibiotics were developed to stop infection and save lives, our bodies were full of great colonies of microorganisms that gobbled up germs and other invading forces.

For example, if the bacteria that causes candida was present in the intestine, these *probiotic* cultures would digest the foreign matter and separate it from the intestinal wall so that it could be flushed from the body through the normal elimination of feces.

Probiotics Need Help

Sadly, since antibiotics have been widely used and abused as the first line of defense against disease, these necessary probiotics are in short supply. Even with proper enzyme activity and digestion, we still need an enormous number of these friendly bacteria strains to guard against the growth of disease-causing bacteria.

More than three pounds of these floras are required for optimal functioning. Some of the best-known strains of these friendly floras are acidophilus, lacto-bacillus, bifidobacterium, and salivarius.

Antibiotics, taken medically, along with those present in our soil, water, and food supply, have reduced the average amount of probiotics available to our bodies to as little as half this. Clearly not enough to keep us young and healthy.

A Breakthrough from Russia

Antibiotic-resistant bacteria have evolved in response to the overprescription of antibiotic drugs, prompting scientists to search for antibiotic alternatives for the treatment of disease. One alternative that is looking very promising is the use of *bacteriophages,* bacteria-eating organisms that live on germs, functioning similarly to probiotics.

Once widely studied, this treatment was cast aside when antibiotics came into favor. The one place where research continued was in the Georgian Republic Children's Hospital in Tbilsi, formerly part of the USSR.

American microbiologists are taking a second look at it as a viable antibiotic alternative.

Prebiotics to the Rescue

Considering all the pressure put on these kindly probiotic bacteria to fend off invasion from the germ warfare waged against our bodies, they need all the help they can get.

This help comes from *prebiotics,* nondigestible carbohydrates that fertilize and nourish the positive strains of bacteria that are battling disease. Look for *Fructo-oligosaccharides* (FOS), a potent prebiotic that tastes like sugar syrup but is not metabolized as sugar and is nonglycemic.

Prebiotics and probiotics working together keep you feeling healthy and energetic—and keep you regular, too. Note: Take them on an empty stomach.

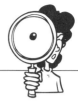

WatchWord

Bacteriophages are viral predators that are among the most common organisms on earth. Like antibiotics, they kill bacteria and germs that could be destructive to the body. They are completely natural and function similarly to probiotics and prebiotics in protecting the body against disease.

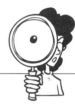

WatchWord

Prebiotics are nondigestible carbohydrates that assist probiotics in promoting the growth of beneficial bacteria in the intestine.

The Least You Need to Know

➤ Depletion of the soil has robbed our food supply of necessary nutrients.

➤ Natural food-based supplements help supply the body with essential vitamins and minerals.

➤ The enzyme-producing capacity of the body diminishes markedly with age.

➤ Taking enzyme supplements and eating raw foods and juices replenishes our enzyme supply.

➤ Prebiotics and probiotics assist digestion, elimination, and cell regeneration.

Part 5

Dear Doctor

Years ago when you thought of your doctor, the immediate image that came to mind was a kindly gentleman in a white lab coat with a stethoscope draped around his neck and a round mirror on a band around his head.

My, times have changed.

For starters, your doctor may be a she, not a he. And the care you receive may be very different from the traditional Western medical mode practiced until the last quarter of the twentieth century.

The practice of medicine isn't all that has changed. We the patients have, too. We are more informed and less willing to turn over control of the care of our health to a single person with the letters "M.D." after his or her name. We are living longer and fuller lives, and we expect our health care to measure up.

You'll learn what your doctor needs to know from you and what you need to know from your doctor. We'll also introduce you to a wealth of alternative health care modalities and tell you about herbs, spices, and essential oils that make your youth quest exciting. Last but not least, we discuss cosmetic surgery and corrective dentistry that radically alter how you look and feel.

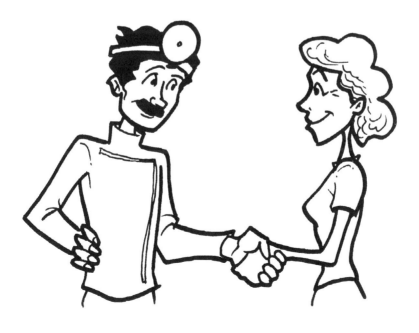

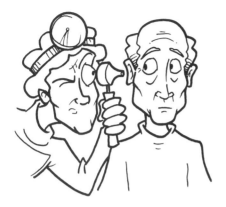

Chapter 21

Health Care to Stay Young

In This Chapter

➤ What we mean by the term "doctor"

➤ How to communicate with your health care practitioner

➤ What to expect from a physical examination

➤ What a good eye exam reveals

By now, you are aware that you can't take your health for granted, especially as you age. The more attention you give to your body, the better you'll look and feel with each passing year.

What's great is that there are a wealth of health care practitioners from a wide range of modalities ready to partner with you in this quest.

This chapter covers what to expect from your physician, your dentist, and your eye doctor. The next chapter, "Widening Your Health Care Horizons," expands your options with acupuncture, chiropractic, massage, meditation, and reflexology.

What We Mean When We Say "Doctor"

Until recently, the word "doctor" referred almost exclusively to graduates of medical schools with specialties in areas like gynecology, family medicine, psychiatry, internal medicine, pediatrics, etc. There were smaller numbers of doctors of osteopathy, chiropractic, homeopathy, and naturopathy.

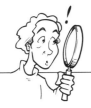

These days, with more than half of Americans seeking alternative forms of health care, that definition has expanded to include a wider range of modalities: traditional Chinese medicine, acupuncture, and Ayurvedic medicine, for example.

Unless we specify a certain discipline, we will be using the term *health care practitioner* and *doctor* interchangeably to cover all of these related modalities.

Age Alert

If you experience any dramatic changes (any change in bladder or bowel habits, unusual rectal discharge or bleeding, prolonged indigestion, persistent hoarseness or nagging cough, a sore throat that won't go away, difficulty swallowing), make note of them and notify your health care practitioner. They may be nothing ... but again, they may mean something serious.

Reveal Your Feelings and Fears

Doctors need to know more than just your name and what's wrong with you before beginning treatment. After all, you live with your concerns, and the doctor only sees you in the office for specified amounts of time.

You are one of the many patients they see in a day, making it even more imperative that you communicate clearly and candidly with them.

Sharing your concerns about aging helps create a warm, productive partnership. The better your doctor knows you, the more sensitively he or she can provide for you.

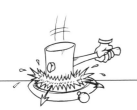

Time Stopper

Fear can age you. If you're experiencing weakness, fatigue, excessive sleeping, a recurring pain (anything that could be a symptom of serious illness or a chronic condition), get it checked. Not knowing can cause more stress and worry than finding out what's going on with your body and treating it accordingly.

Making the Right Match

Look for a doctor like you would look for a best friend. The fit has to be right.

You can't tell by the diplomas on the wall, the address, or the decor of the waiting room. You'll have to tap into your feelings. If something doesn't feel right, it probably isn't. This doesn't mean that there's anything wrong with the practitioner, only that this one's not right for you.

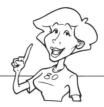

Voice of Experience

"The Doctor of the Future will give no medicine, but will interest his patients in the Care of the Human frame, in diet, and in the cause and prevention of disease."

—Thomas Alva Edison

Choosing someone to be your partner in staying healthy and young is a highly personal matter. Trust your instincts and follow them.

What Your Doctor Wants to Know

Your doctor needs to know a great deal about you and your family history, especially if it's your first visit.

Dr. Dana G. Cohen, director of New York's Center for Complementary and Internal Medicine, has a five-page form she asks patients to complete to give her a firm foundation for planning that patient's care.

"I spend an hour on that first appointment," she explains. "I want more than the patient's medical history—past hospitalizations, illnesses, health of their parents and grandparents. I also take a social history—smoking, alcohol, marital status, exercise."

Dr. Cohen is one of a new breed of doctors who has extensive knowledge of nutrition and age-reversing breakthroughs. The more a physician is aware of current research, the more he or she will be able to guide you in your quest for youth.

In addition to the obvious (name, address, telephone numbers, e-mail address, date of birth, age,

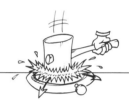

Time Stopper

Have you ever gone into your doctor's office with a long list of questions in your head, only to have them fly out the window the moment you open your mouth? All of a sudden, everything's a blur. What's the solution? Write everything down.

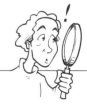

Age Alert

Don't hold anything back. You can't say anything that will shock your health care practitioner. The secrets you keep will impede your care.

sex, and marital status), Dr. Cohen wants to know what the patient does for a living and how long he or she has been in that job.

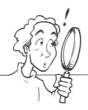

She also asks that patients list, as concisely as possible, the main reasons, in order of importance, that spurred them to seek medical attention. "Sometimes that gets lost in the process of taking the patient's history," she explains. This also sheds light on what the patient feels needs attention.

Dr. Cohen's assessment form is so inclusive, we're passing it along in slightly modified form so that you can be prepared to meet with your own physician. By providing complete and accurate answers to each of these questions, you'll be helping your health care practitioner fully understand your medical history and risk factors. This can make a big difference in your treatment program.

Age Alert

It's important not to be intimidated and to take your time to thoroughly discuss everything—since the doctor's working for *you.*

Health Assessment Form

Medications

Please list all medications that you currently take, their strength, and how often.

This list should include not just the medications your doctor has prescribed. List any over-the-counter drugs, like aspirin and ibuprofen, cold and flu medications, decongestants, antacids—anything you take on a self-determined, as-needed basis.

What is your current weight? _____ Your ideal weight? _____

What is the most you have ever weighed? _____

The least? _____

Habits

Do you currently smoke? _____ If yes, what? _____

How much? _____ For how long? _____

Have you ever smoked? _____ If yes, how much? _____

If yes, when did you quit? _____ Do you chew tobacco? _____

Do you currently drink alcohol? _____

If so, what and how often? ("Socially" is not an acceptable answer.)

_____

Have you ever had a drinking problem? _____

If yes, how long have you been sober? _____

Do you regularly attend addiction support group meetings? _____

Which? _____

Do you use drugs in a recreational way? _____

If so, which ones? _____

Have you ever used intravenous drugs? _____

If so, when was the last time? _____

Have you ever been treated for drug abuse? _____

Do you still regularly get treatment for this problem? _____

If yes, what? _____

Exercise

Do you currently exercise? _____

If so, what do you do?   How often?

_____   _____

_____   _____

_____   _____

Miscellaneous

How many hours of sleep do you get each night? _____

Do you feel rested in the morning? _____

Can you remember your dreams? _____

Are you sexually active? _____

Do you use condoms during sexual intercourse? _____

Vitamins and Supplements

Please list all vitamins and supplements that you take on a regular basis, including strength and how taken. (Include vitamins, nutritional supplements, herbal compounds, etc.)

Vitamin/Supplement	Strength	Taken
_____	_____	_____
_____	_____	_____
_____	_____	_____

[Note: Dr. Cohen's form has 21 spaces, indicating her awareness in the use of vitamins and supplements.]

Allergies

Please list any known allergies to medications, foods, or environmental substances.

_____	_____	_____
_____	_____	_____

Medical History

Please list any hospitalizations (including childbirth):

_____

continues

221

continued

Please list any surgeries you have had (including childbirth):

_____

Please list any major illnesses you currently have or have had in the past:

_____

Are you presently under the care of a physician? _____
If so, whom? _____
Address: _____
Phone number: _____

Dietary Habits

How many times per day/week do you eat the following foods?

Beef _____   Chicken _____   Fish _____
Pork _____   Other _____   Eggs _____
Cheese _____   Vegetables _____   Salads _____
Fruits _____   Sugar (cake/candy/ice cream, etc.) _____

What do you drink with your meals? _____
What do you drink in between meals? _____ How many times per day/week do you eat the following foods?

Beef _____   Chicken _____   Fish _____
Pork _____   Other _____   Eggs _____
Cheese _____   Vegetables _____   Salads _____
Fruits _____   Sugar (cake/candy/ice cream, etc.) _____

What do you drink with your meals? _____
What do you drink in between meals? _____

Please list what you would normally eat in a given day:
Breakfast: _____
Lunch: _____
Dinner: _____
Snacks: _____

Psychological Assessment

Do you experience cloudy thinking? _____
Do you consider yourself under stress? _____
How much does stress interfere with your life? _____
Are you under stress at home? _____ If so, why? _____
Are you under stress at work? _____ If so, why? _____
Do you become frequently depressed? _____
Have you ever been treated for depression? _____

If so, how? _____

Do you have wide mood swings? _____

Do you consider yourself compulsive? _____

Do you consider yourself impulsive? _____

Can you let off steam easily? _____

Are you anxious? _____

Do you get riled easily? _____

Health Maintenance

When was your last complete physical exam? _____

Have you ever had a sigmoidoscopy or colonoscopy? _____

If so, When? _____ Result _____

Reason for exam: _____

Have you ever had an EKG? _____ If so, when? _____

Have you ever had a stress test? _____ If so, when? _____

Have you ever had a tuberculosis test? _____

If so, when? _____

Have you ever received the BCG vaccine? _____

Have you ever had a chest x-ray? _____ If so, when? _____

Result: _____ Reason for exam: _____

Men:

Have you ever had a prostate examination? _____

If so, when? _____ Results: _____

Have you had a PSA blood test? _____ If so, when? _____

Results: _____

Do you regularly examine your testicles for lumps? _____

Women:

Do you regularly examine your breasts for lumps? _____

Have you had a mammogram? _____ If so, when? _____

Results: _____

Have you had a pap smear? _____ If so, when? _____

Results: _____

Family History

Is your mother still alive? _____ If so, what is her age? _____

If not, what was her cause of death? _____

Did/Does she have any medical conditions? _____

Please describe: _____

Is your father still alive? _____ If so, what is his age? _____

If not, what was his cause of death? _____

continues

continued

Did/Does he have any medical conditions? _____
Please describe: _____
Do you have any siblings? _____ What are their ages? _____
Please list their name(s) and medical conditions, if any:

_____

Has anyone in your family had or do they have any of the following conditions?

Relationship_____	**Relationship**
Diabetes _____	Obesity_____
Cancer_____	Heart attack_____
High blood pressure _____	Stroke _____
Asthma _____	Eczema _____
Thyroid disease _____	Osteoporosis _____

Adapted from the form used by Dr. Dana G. Cohen.

Your Body, Head to Toe

At first glance, some of this may seem repetitious. This review reminds you of conditions you may have forgotten or tolerated so long they have become "normal."

Review of Body Systems

	Present	Past
Skin		
Skin growths	_____	_____
Change in color of growth	_____	_____
Skin cancer	_____	_____
Hives	_____	_____
Rashes	_____	_____
Athlete's foot	_____	_____
Hair loss	_____	_____
Nail fungus	_____	_____
Respiratory		
Shortness of breath	_____	_____
Wheezing	_____	_____
Chronic cough	_____	_____
Blood in sputum	_____	_____
Bronchitis	_____	_____

	Present	Past
Emphysema	_____	_____
Pneumonia	_____	_____
Asthma	_____	_____

Genito-Urinary

	Present	Past
Nausea	_____	_____
Vomiting	_____	_____
Abdominal pains	_____	_____
Heartburn	_____	_____
Recurring diarrhea	_____	_____
Frequent constipation	_____	_____
Changes in bowel habit	_____	_____
Blood in stool	_____	_____
Black stool	_____	_____
Gallstones	_____	_____
Ulcers	_____	_____
Hepatitis (which type?)	_____	_____

Neurologic

	Present	Past
Recurrent headaches	_____	_____
Migraine headaches	_____	_____
Dizziness	_____	_____
Speech difficulties	_____	_____
Visual disturbances	_____	_____
Muscle weakness	_____	_____
Memory loss	_____	_____
Seizures	_____	_____

Cardiovascular

	Present	Past
Chest pains	_____	_____
Palpitations	_____	_____
Murmurs	_____	_____
Heart attack	_____	_____
Rheumatic fever	_____	_____
High blood pressure	_____	_____
Irregular heartbeats	_____	_____
Atrial fibrillation	_____	_____
Fainting	_____	_____
Ankle swelling	_____	_____
Leg pain while walking	_____	_____

continues

Review of Body Systems   (continued)

	Present	Past
Ear/Nose/Throat		
Wear glasses or contacts	_____	_____
Double vision	_____	_____
Cataracts	_____	_____
Eye pain	_____	_____
Color blindness	_____	_____
Hearing loss	_____	_____
Ringing in the ears	_____	_____
Ear pain	_____	_____
Sinus problems	_____	_____
Nosebleeds	_____	_____
Decreased ability to smell	_____	_____
Frequent sore throats	_____	_____
Hoarseness	_____	_____
Difficulty swallowing	_____	_____

Gynecological

Age of menstrual onset _____	Age of menopause _____
Interval between periods _____	Duration of periods (days) _____
Painful menstruation _____	Last menstrual period _____
Regular periods _____	
Number of pregnancies _____	Number of live births _____
Number of miscarriages _____	Number of abortions _____
Hormone replacement _____	Birth-control pills _____
Gestational diabetes _____	

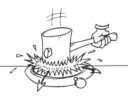

Time Stopper

Memo to women over 40: Ask your physician for a Pyrilinks–D test. This urine test measures your rate of bone loss. At 50, ask for a bone-density test, and do this periodically.

Listen Up

Often forgotten but not to be overlooked is hearing.

You may not notice that you've been turning up the sound on the TV or asking people to repeat themselves. If you find yourself saying, "What ...?" it's time to have your hearing tested.

New, almost invisible hearing aids are available. Don't be ashamed to get one if you need it.

The Eyes Have It

Changes in vision are one of the first things we notice with aging. We find ourselves squinting at the TV or holding the newspaper at arm's length. Before long, we break down and have our eyes checked. Will we need bifocals (like Grandpa) or just a pair of reading specs? Only an eye exam will tell.

You can consult with an *optometrist* or *ophthalmologist* for such an exam. Both can check your vision and the health of your eyes, but only an ophthalmologist can perform surgery and prescribe drugs.

What the Eye Doctor Sees

An examination of the eyes checks more than your vision. Optometrist Dr. Allan Cohen of Eye to Eye Vision Center in New York City advises yearly exams after the age of 40.

Since eye care involves more than how well you see or don't see, this exam will involve tests for a series of possible problems:

➤ **Glaucoma** is a common and severe disorder that, left untreated, can lead to blindness. Diagnosed only by testing the fluid pressure in the eye, symptoms may be headaches and loss of peripheral vision. Glaucoma is easily treated with drops or surgery to lower pressure.

➤ **Cataracts** are opaque and cloudy areas occurring in the normally clear lens of the eye that may block or distort light and progressively reduce vision. Early diagnosis is possible during a complete examination of the eye. In an advanced cataract, a misty circular area is visible within the pupil, which normally appears black. Cataracts are treatable with surgery.

Age Alert

When preparing to see your doctor, make a list of every medication—prescription and otherwise— you take. *Note:* Birth-control pills and hormone-replacement therapy are medicines. List them, too.

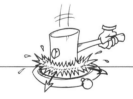

Time Stopper

At 40, all men should have a base-line PSA blood test. This screens for *prostate-specific antigen,* which is indicative of potential prostate cancer. This is especially important if you are African American or you have a family history of cancer, warns Dr. Dana G. Cohen.

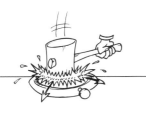

Time Stopper

Everyone—man or woman—over the age of 50 should be examined for colon cancer and other intestinal disorders. One way this is done is by a flexible sigmoidoscopy exam. In addition, stool samples should be tested yearly for occult blood (which can only be detected by a microscopic or chemical analysis).

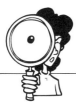

WatchWord

Optometrists are trained and licensed to test vision and prescribe corrective lenses. **Ophthalmologists** are medical doctors who specialize in diseases and surgery of the eyes.

What the Retina Reveals

It's amazing what a practiced professional eye can see by looking at the cornea, lens, fluids, and optic disc and nerves. Even diseases totally unrelated to the eye show up.

Dr. Cohen says, "By looking at the back of the eye, the retina, we can see evidence of high blood pressure, diabetes … sometimes even brain tumors." When this happens, he refers his patients to an ophthalmologist or internist for treatment.

Bifocals, Anyone?

Hardly anyone over 40 escapes the need of some form of corrective lenses. Most common are bifocals.

"Bifocals" describes the kind of lens where you can see a line or circle. The prescription for distance is in the top part of the lens, with the near-vision prescription cut into the lower part. This can give an unattractive, aged look to your face.

Try the more advanced "progressive lens" with no visible line. The correction is multifocal, gradually changing from top to bottom. Besides looking better than conventional bifocals, the correction is superior.

And if you prefer not to wear glasses at all, you might try contact lenses. Bifocal prescriptions are available in soft, gas-permeable, and hard lenses. The near-vision prescription on the bottom of the lens is slightly heavier, which keeps the contacts in place.

Once, as Hattie was doing exercises with her bifocal contact lenses, she bent over to do a hamstring stretch. When she stood up, her vision was distorted. After a few moments, the heavier part of the lens slipped back into place, and all was well again. "A minor handicap, considering how great they are," she laughs.

The Least You Need to Know

➤ The word "doctor" has expanded to include a wide range of Western and Eastern modalities.

➤ Being open with your doctor when it comes to your concerns about aging helps establish the best course of action.

➤ A comprehensive physical exam takes into account not just your health history but your family's as well.

➤ Your hearing should be checked periodically, because hearing loss is a common consequence of aging.

➤ Have a full eye exam every year.

➤ Eye surgery can correct nearsightedness.

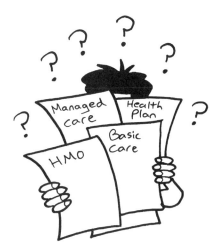

Chapter 22

Widening Your Health Care Horizons

In This Chapter

➤ Using alternatives to traditional Western medicine

➤ Learning the importance of massage

➤ Understanding chiropractic, osteopathy, and homeopathy

➤ Practicing health care in the Chinese tradition

➤ Exploring complementary modalities

We Americans seem to have our hands full when it comes to chronic disease. Conditions like heart disease, diabetes, arthritis, asthma, allergies, immune disorders, and cancer—the list goes on—were considered to be unavoidable consequences of aging.

We strongly disagree.

It's not age that causes poor health. It's the number of years people have subjected their bodies to inadequate and even shabby care.

Staying superbly youthful and healthy can be daunting. No wonder it's achieved by so few. With work and family pressures, it's hard to go it alone. But you don't have to.

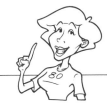

Voice of Experience

When health is absent, wisdom cannot reveal itself, art cannot manifest, strength cannot fight, wealth becomes useless, and joy cannot be felt.

—Herophilies, physician to Alexander the Great (300 B.C.E.)

Where to Turn

Diet and exercise, teamed with routine medical exams, has often been the only option available for health-conscious Americans. This is no longer true. An increasing number of alternatives to orthodox *allopathic* Western medical practices are proving to be highly effective.

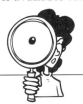

WatchWord

Mainstream Western doctors routinely fight disease by **allopathic** means. They rely on technology, focusing on the physical body, generally excluding the effects of the mind, body, and spirit.

Nowadays, regardless of where you live, you will be able to find highly qualified practitioners of most of these complementary disciplines to partner with you. Adding chiropractic, acupuncture, and several other modalities to your arsenal further extends your options. Some, like meditation, yoga, and massage, though not specifically medical, have a strong therapeutic value that makes them worthy of consideration.

They've proven their worth through centuries of use.

We're starting with massage as a simple first step to alternative healing.

In Touch with Massage

There is no denying that we all are under continuous stress, and stress creates even more stress. How do we break this vicious cycle? One powerful way is with massage.

Every baby gets massaged several times a day—when diapered, bathed, held. We adults, by sharp contrast, take a fast shower, dress, and basically forget about our bodies. The body doesn't like this neglect and retaliates with sickness, exhaustion, lack of sexuality, and a generalized dullness. All these symptoms can be reversed markedly with massage.

We recommend that you have a massage as often as your budget allows. It's one of the best things you can do for yourself. It's luxurious and healing at the same time … a luxury that's a necessity.

Everyone Benefits

We assert that everyone benefits from massage, not just an athlete with a pulled hamstring or a wealthy woman indulging her senses at a spa. Massage not only increases circulation, it also helps erase chronic and acute discomfort and increase flexibility.

Licensed massage therapist Joel Benjamin, whose client list reads like a who's who of New York theater and dance circles, notes that "Loss of flexibility is one of the most insidious signs of aging."

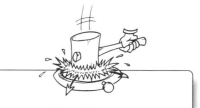

Time Stopper

As we grow older, our circulation becomes more sluggish. It is critical to encourage the blood to move through places where stress and tension are stored. The upper shoulders and back are especially vulnerable.

How Massage Retards Aging

A former dancer himself, Joel adds that regular massage is beneficial in retarding the aging process both in mind and body:

Massage stimulates circulation, taking blood through the body, to the limbs, toes, and fingers, and even lowers blood pressure. And with more blood going to your brain, you'll be more alert.

What's more, since it stimulates the production of endorphins, it eases depression and improves your feeling of well-being.

Different Strokes

Several types of massage are in general use. If at all possible, we suggest that you try them all to decide which works best for you and your body.

Says Joel, "Massage allows for nonsexual, nonthreatening touch. It takes us back to the natural human need to be nurtured."

Here are some of the widely available types of massage:

➤ **Swedish massage.** This anatomy-based system of massage uses five kinds of strokes, each defined by how they work on the muscles, nerves, and lymphatic system.

Effleurage consists of soothing strokes along the length of the muscles.

233

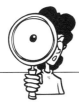

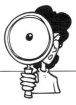

Petrissage is stimulating strokes, rubbing against the grain of the muscles.

Friction consists of rubbing muscles against the bone, usually at the joint, to release deep knots in the muscles.

Vibration calls for stimulating and soothing moves that relieve tension and increase circulation.

Tapotement is a series of percussive strikes that relieve pain.

➤ **Acupressure.** Using the fingers and hands instead of needles, acupressure, like acupuncture, stimulates the thousands of meridians along which life energy, or *qi,* flows.

➤ **Shiatsu.** Like acupressure, this Japanese massage technique uses the meridians, or acupressure points, throughout the body to guide the therapist's touch.

➤ **Reiki.** A Tibetan discipline, Reiki practitioners channel energy into the client's body by placing their hands over specific parts of the body.

➤ **Trigger-point massage.** The therapist concentrates on massaging any weakened points within the muscles to release pain and strengthen the muscle tissue.

➤ **Deep-tissue massage.** Similar to trigger-point work, this technique deeply manipulates the muscles. This can be uncomfortable, even painful, but the results will be long-lasting.

➤ **Lymphatic drainage.** This technique concentrates on the lymph system, helping the body to eliminate wastes and toxins.

➤ *Reflexology.* This technique begins with the feet. The therapist uses thumb and forefinger to stimulate the areas of the feet that correspond to specific areas of the body. This is known as *zone therapy* in England.

➤ **Rolfing.** A program of deep-tissue massage designed to correct the body's alignment and posture by releasing tension and trauma in the fascia or connective tissue.

➤ **Alexander Technique.** Practitioners of this technique use gentle strokes to correct distortions in posture. They concentrate on improving overall posture, which they say is the source of all sorts of disorders, including tension and pain, respiratory and muscular problems, and hormonal imbalances.

➤ **Feldenkrais Method.** Gentle healing touch teams with movement training, awareness, and psychological dialogue to release tension and pain in the body.

We've given massage a lot of attention so that you can be completely familiar with its benefits. The other complementary disciplines we'll profile next will give you a taste of some modalities that are also available to you.

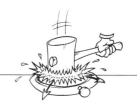

Time Stopper

When you go to a chiropractor, don't be afraid of the sounds you hear emanating from your body when it's being adjusted. The popping sound isn't a bone breaking. It simply indicates that pressure is being released in the joint.

Chiropractic and Osteopathy Get Back to Basics

These two disciplines are so well-known they can hardly be considered "alternative modalities." Many people use them to complement the treatment they receive from their primary care physician.

Both chiropractors and *osteopaths* treat the body by manually adjusting the joints, particularly the vertebrae of the spine. By focused pressure, they release tension and adjust misalignments. Correcting these mechanical disorders increases blood and lymph circulation and stimulates nerve activity, thereby encouraging healing.

Chiropractors often recommend vitamins and supplements but cannot prescribe medication. Osteopaths are medical doctors and therefore can write prescriptions.

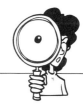

WatchWord

Osteopathy is the medical practice that incorporates manipulation of the bones to treat ailments which they believe result from the pressure of displaced bones on nerves.

"Like Cures Like"—Homeopathy

Homeopathy, a complete system of complementary medicine based on the principle that "like cures like," was developed by a German physician, Samuel Hahnemann (1755–1843). He formulated medicines that create a condition that is similar to the illness, causing the body to defend itself against the pathology. As the body's defenses are activated, they work to cure the disease.

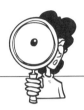

WatchWord

Homeopathy is a complete system of complementary medicine based on the principle that "like cures like." Homeopathic remedies stimulate the body's defenses to cure disease.

Traditional Chinese Medicine

To the Chinese, health is a state of balance and wholeness, in which all parts of the body, mind, and spirit are in harmony.

Behind this thinking is the acknowledgement that all of reality is composed of paradoxical opposites called *yin* and *yang.* Everything has two sides—good and bad, front and back, left and right—and all of life is a struggle to maintain balance, or harmony, between these opposites. All illness stems from imbalance of something in the person's life.

This healing tradition combines herbalism, using specially prepared healing foods to achieve balance, acupuncture, and a variety of other therapeutic practices, such as *qi kung,* to maintain the body in health and harmony.

Acupuncture Gets to the Point

A component of traditional Chinese medicine that is finding acceptance in the West, acupuncture is the placement of fine needles into the body at specific points along the *meridians* to treat specific health problems so that all organs and tissues receive the energy needed for the body to function optimally.

Two Thousand Years of Practice

Acupuncture has evolved over 2000 years and has been deemed suitable for treating a variety of conditions by the World Health Organization. These

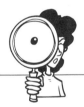

WatchWord

An ancient Chinese healing exercise discipline, **qi kung**—energy work—combines slow, precise movements; powerful, controlled breathing; and sounds that remove energy blockages and increase the flow of blood and qi to all vital organs.

conditions include toothaches, pain after extraction, earaches, sinus inflammation, respiratory disorders such as bronchial asthma, inflammation of the colon, constipation, and diarrhea.

Acupuncture is also widely used to relieve headaches, including migraines, nerve pain, aches from sprains, lower back pain, stiffness in the joints, and osteoarthritis.

Releasing Shock Waves

"We must look at the body as a whole," explains Florence Patsy Roth, L.Ac. "An accident, for example, causes many layers of shock to the body. The body reacts to trauma in a very protective way. To keep from being hurt any more, it tightens up, producing muscle tension and energy blockages. Acupuncture can release these tensions so that the body is more flexible and balanced."

With respect to looking and feeling younger, Patsy notes, "Increased blood and lymph circulation, as well as movement of energy, promotes a feeling of balance. That in itself gives you a better sense of well-being."

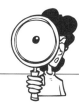

WatchWord

Meridians are channels throughout the body through which qi—energy—flows. Energy blockages at the points where the meridians intersect can be released through acupuncture and acupressure massage.

Consider These Options, Too

Believe it or not, what we Americans consider traditional Western medicine is one of the new kids on the block when it comes to healing and health care.

Consider exploring several other healing philosophies that can provide youth-enhancing energy and spiritual enlightenment. They are becoming increasingly popular and are being offered through adult educational programs and community centers. Give them a try. This should keep you busy for a while.

➤ **Yoga.** Yoga works with postures to achieve harmony of mind and body. It incorporates breathing, visualization, and exercises that stretch and strengthen the musculature. There are several types of yoga, each with a different emphasis. These disciplines are proving to be quite valuable in countering stress.

➤ **Meditation.** This involves being aware of breathing and repeating a *mantra* for deep mental focus. Its object is the achievement of total relaxation and clarity of mind.

➤ **Visualization.** This technique involves focusing on ideas or images to paint an optimistic, life-affirming picture in your mind. These images can be used as an antidote to repetitive, morbid thoughts.

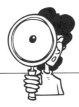

➤ **Neurolinguistic programming.** NLP is a technique based on the assumption that the body and mind are connected. It teaches you how to reframe your thinking patterns and ultimately to take alternate actions to break habits.

➤ **Biofeedback.** This process uses a mechanism strapped to the body to measure increased sweating, pulse, and muscle tension. As you monitor your reactions, you can develop effective ways of reducing stress.

➤ **Hypnotherapy.** In this therapy, you are placed in a trance state to implant positive messages for relieving addiction, habits, anxiety, phobias, and pain.

➤ **Bach Flower Remedies.** Derived from wildflowers diluted in pure water and coded to specific conditions, these compounds were invented by Dr. Edward Bach around the turn of the twentieth century. They are now used extensively. The most common is Rescue Remedy, a combination of five flower extracts, to treat anxiety.

➤ **Bates Method for Eyesight.** This therapy asserts that most vision defects arise from tension and poor function of the muscles controlling the lens. The Bates Method provides exercises to strengthen these muscles.

➤ **Hydrotherapy.** This therapy uses the relaxing, rejuvenating power of water to stimulate the circulation, nourish injured or diseased areas of the body, and eliminate toxins.

➤ **Antigravity therapy.** By doing yoga-style headstands or using a mechanical apparatus that supports the body and relieves pressure on the head and neck, you increase the blood circulation to your brain, which improves memory, vision, hearing, complexion, hair growth, and gum health. Also known as inversion therapy.

➤ **Chelation therapy.** A form of medical treatment using intravenous solutions containing minerals, vitamins and a special amino acid—ethylene diamine tetracetic acid (EDTA)—to remove toxic heavy metals such as lead, mercury, and arsenic from the body and to reverse hardening of the arteries.

The Least You Need to Know

➤ There are many alternatives to allopathic or traditional medicine.

➤ Massage is one of the easiest and most effective ways to relieve stress.

➤ Homeopathy, chiropractic, and osteopathy are the most common forms of complementary health care.

➤ Traditional Chinese medicine, which includes acupuncture and acupressure, is gaining acceptance in the West.

➤ Choosing the modalities that suit your needs is a fascinating adventure in well-being.

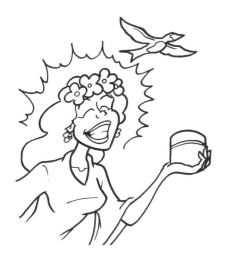

Chapter 23

Mother Nature Has the Answers

In This Chapter

➤ Incorporating healing plants into your life

➤ Directory of therapeutic foods, herbs, and spices

➤ Water—essential for health and youth

➤ Aromatherapy—a rediscovered art

➤ Essential oils and their properties

In Part 4, "Putting Youth on Your Plate," we said you're as young as you eat. That explained how what you eat every day can make the difference between whether you remain young and healthy or old and ill before your time.

Now we're expanding that to make you aware of specific plants, herbs, spices, and essential oils that have magnificent healing properties. You may be using some of them already—in food or around your home—without even realizing their health-giving powers.

Since Time Began

Since Adam and Eve first walked in the Garden of Eden, humans have been curious about their surroundings, tasting and trying everything and recording their reactions. If something tasted pleasant and made them feel good, or cured an ailment, they remembered that. The next time they had an upset stomach, or some other ache and pain, they went back to that plant and consumed it again.

The entire Chinese medical tradition is based on herbs and their uses, as is the Ayurvedic approach from India. According to American Indian mythology, the Great Spirit and Mother Earth told the wise ones—medicine men—which plants, seeds, and roots to use for healing.

Trial, Error, and Truth

According to traditional Chinese medicine, a good doctor is one whose patients are never sick. These healers treated all patients with concoctions formulated to bring balance to the body to keep it well and strong.

Similar methods are recorded in other healing traditions and in the Bible, which lists hundreds of plants with curative powers.

The experiences of these early practitioners of the healing arts survive today, enriching our lives with health and youth-giving care.

In the Body, in the Home

The life-enhancing properties of these plants extend beyond their use in food. They can be brewed into teas, used in poultices, and even mixed into cleaning preparations for the home.

A garden of fragrant plants and even a fresh bouquet of flowers indoors can have a calming or uplifting effect on one's spirits.

Besides providing a lovely glow, scented candles create a mood in the home that relaxes and soothes even the most stressed among us.

Foods, Herbs, and Spices for Life

That basil in your spaghetti sauce does more than taste good. It's a nerve tonic that is slightly antiseptic, relieves nausea and headaches, and increases lactation in nursing mothers.

The cinnamon you sprinkled on your applesauce and cappuccino stimulates digestion, promotes circulation, freshens your breath, and soothes away toothache pain.

And what about garlic? It's a veritable pharmacy. A potent detoxifier, it rivals many an antibiotic in its healing properties.

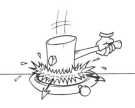

Time Stopper

The National Institutes of Health reports that national sales of botanical dietary supplements—including herbal compounds, extracts, and teas—exceed $1.5 billion a year and are increasing annually by 25 percent.

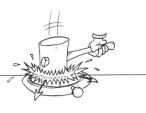

Time Stopper

Drop a tiny bit of oil of lavender on a light bulb. The heat of the bulb diffuses this uplifting essence into your room.

Isn't it nice to know that in addition to tasting great, these herbs and spices contribute to your health and youth?

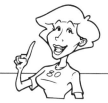

Voice of Experience

Gautam Mukerji, general manager of New York's Bay Leaf restaurant, instructs us on food and Indian spices: "Indian spices play a major role in the well-being of the human anatomy as they help to cleanse the body of all its toxins and wastes. Indian food can help the Western world by showing it how to use spices to enhance the quality of life."

Here's a list of several plant-based foods, herbs, and spices. Some may already be on your spice rack. Others, such as maca, chanca piedra, and camu-camu, have been around for centuries but only recently have come to our attention.

➤ **Anise seeds.** These have a mild licorice taste. They work as a digestive aid, help respiratory infections, alleviate menopausal symptoms, and promote milk production in nursing mothers.

➤ **Astralagus.** This is used as an energy and heart tonic. It regulates blood pressure and blood sugar, improves circulation, boosts the immune system, and helps heal wounds.

➤ **Basil.** This slightly antiseptic "nerve tonic" fights anxiety, relieves nausea and headaches, and stimulates lactation in nursing mothers.

➤ **Chanca piedra.** Also known as "break-stone," this South American herb breaks up and expels kidney stones and gallstones. It promotes healthy liver and gall bladder functions, and it clears obstructions of internal organs. It also treats edema, excess uric acid, constipation, dysentery, and stomachaches.

➤ **Camu-camu.** This provides antiviral and analgesic properties. It's especially good for migraines and can be used as an antidepressant.

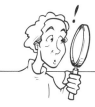

Age Alert

Remember that herbs and spices, when used medicinally, are very potent. They may seem innocent enough, but if misused, they can be dangerous. Make sure to follow directions in preparation, dosage, and particularly, frequency. You want to be sure they are helping rather than harming you.

It's effective against herpes and vaginal yeast infections. Camu-camu contains more vitamin C than any other known plant.

➤ **Cat's claw.** This is used to cleanse the intestinal tract. It eases stomach and bowel disorders and helps with diverticulitis, colitis, hemorrhoids, gastritis, ulcers, parasites, and intestinal flora imbalance.

➤ **Cayenne.** These hot, spicy pepper seeds can stimulate digestion, increase circulation, and ward off colds and sore throats. Cayenne is also good for the heart, kidneys, lungs, arthritis, and rheumatism.

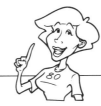

Voice of Experience

Nutritionist Joy Pierson, co-owner with Bart Potenza of New York's award-winning vegan restaurant the Candle Café, offers a potent health drink.

Joy's Immune-Booster Cocktail

½ teaspoon cayenne

1 tablespoon fresh ginger juice

2 tablespoons fresh lemon juice

1 ounce apple juice

½ teaspoon honey

6 ounces hot water

Stir, drink, and get well.

➤ **Celery.** An antioxidant with sedative properties, celery helps reduce blood pressure, relieves muscle spasms, and improves the appetite.

➤ **Carrots.** Carrots are high in beta-carotene and work as an antioxidant. They're good for cleansing the liver and the skin.

➤ **Cinnamon.** Cinnamon promotes circulation, eases rheumatic pain, sweetens the breath, and lessens heavy menstrual flow.

➤ **Echinacea.** This immune-system booster commonly is used to treat the symptoms of colds, sore throats, and flu.

➤ **Fennel.** This is an anise-like flavored digestive aid and appetite suppressant. It works as a breath freshener; clears the lungs; and relieves abdominal pain, stomach spasms, bloating, and gas.

➤ **Garlic.** A major detoxifier and natural antibiotic, garlic boosts the immune system, eases arteriosclerosis and circulatory problems, and works as an antiseptic.

➤ **Ginkgo biloba.** This antioxidant increases blood flow to the brain, improves the memory, and improves hearing loss.

➤ **Ginger root.** Ginger root is an antispasmodic, antibacterial, antimicrobial, and antioxidant. It treats bowel disorders, helps circulatory problems, relieves indigestion, and settles an upset stomach.

➤ **Goldenseal.** Also called "orangeroot," this functions as an antiseptic and a stomach tonic. It helps adrenal glands and eases stress, anxiety, and nervousness. It's also used to treat asthma and allergies. Goldenseal is toxic in large doses; use it for no longer than a week. Pregnant women should not use goldenseal.

➤ **Green tea.** This tea contains numerous antioxidant compounds, lowers cholesterol levels, helps regulate blood sugar and insulin levels, and combats mental fatigue. Limit the intake of green tea if you are pregnant or have anxiety disorders.

➤ **Kelp.** Kelp is important for brain tissue and nerve development. Its high iodine content is helpful in treating thyroid and mineral deficiencies. Kelp strengthens nails and blood vessels and can be used as a salt substitute.

➤ **Maca.** Maca helps regulate the endocrine glands—adrenals, thyroid, pancreas, ovaries, and testes. It supports and balances estrogen and progesterone levels in women and testosterone levels in men. Maca regulates menstruation and eases PMS. It also has been proven to be safe and effective as an alternative to hormone replacement therapy (*HRT*).

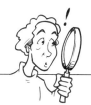

Age Alert

Premarin, the most commonly prescribed estrogen-replacement drug, gets its name from the pregnant mare urine that is used in its manufacture. Are you aware that the animals that provide the urine receive painful, inhumane treatment? Explore the many safe, effective varieties of plant-based HRT.

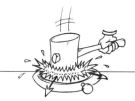

Time Stopper

Don't think of parsley as merely a garnish. It contains more vitamin C per weight than oranges—and freshens your breath, too.

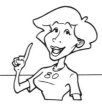

Voice of Experience

According to Viana Muller, Ph.D., an anthropologist who first imported this amazing herbal supplement to this country, "The maca root is a medicinal herb from Peru that stimulates the ovaries and adrenals into working better. Maca helps postmenopausal women who suffer from vaginal dryness and loss of libido to have adequate vaginal lubrication and to 'get in the mood' again."

➤ **Milk thistle.** This strong liver cleanser is helpful in treating poison ivy and works as an immune-system booster.

➤ **Mint.** This category includes peppermint, spearmint, and wintergreen. It's used as a digestive aid; relieves nausea; stimulates the appetite; relieves diarrhea, headaches, fever, and chills; and works as a breath freshener.

➤ **Mustard seeds.** These improve digestion and aid in the metabolism of fat. They can cause skin irritation if applied directly to the skin. Mustard seeds relieve chest congestion, inflammation from injuries, and joint pain.

➤ **Oregano.** This is an antifungal that is helpful in combating yeast and candida infections.

➤ **Papaya.** Papaya eases heartburn, indigestion, and inflammatory bowel disorders. It also stimulates the appetite.

➤ **Parsley.** Parsley freshens the breath; works as a digestive aid and mild diuretic; and is helpful in treating prostate disorders, gas, and regulating blood pressure. Juiced parsley can clear urinary tract infections.

➤ **Red raspberry.** This relieves cramps, morning sickness, hot flashes, and diarrhea. It also regulates menstrual flow and is helpful in treating canker sores. It's good for the bones, nails, teeth, and skin.

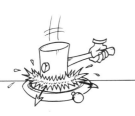

Time Stopper

Powerful medications to treat depression are being prescribed in higher numbers than ever before. Many have unwanted side-effects like weight gain and sexual dysfunction. St. John's Wort, used for centuries, can be a safe, effective alternative. Many people report its success in treating mood swings, **seasonal affective disorder** (**SAD**), and depression.

246

➤ **Rosemary.** This is an antibacterial, astringent, and decongestant. It stimulates circulation and works as a blood-pressure equalizer. Rosemary also treats headaches and menstrual cramps.

➤ **Sage.** Sage stimulates digestion and works as a phytoestrogen that reduces hot flashes. It's beneficial for disorders of the mouth and throat, and it works as an antibiotic. As a rinse, it stimulates hair growth and adds shine.

➤ **Soy.** Soy is rich in the phytoestrogen iso-flavone and may reduce the risk of breast cancer and other reproductive organ cancers. Soy reduces menopausal hot flashes, increases bone density, and develops muscle mass. Soy is high in protein.

➤ **Spirulina.** This is a naturally digestible, highly nutritional microalgae. It helps with mineral-absorption and treats blood-sugar levels for hypoglycemics.

➤ **St. John's Wort.** This strong revitalizer works as a mood uplifter and is widely used in treating depression.

➤ **Thyme.** Thyme is a strong antiseptic that reduces fever and eliminates flatulence. It also lowers cholesterol levels, relieves headaches and liver disease, and stops scalp itch.

➤ **Tumeric.** This is an antibiotic, antioxidant, anti-inflammatory agent. It protects the liver from toxins, increases bone density, and lowers cholesterol.

➤ **Wheatgrass.** This antioxidant is rich in trace minerals. It boosts the immune system and oxygenates the blood. Drinking wheatgrass juice has been known to restore hair color. One caveat: because of its intense cleansing properties, you must follow one shot of wheatgrass juice with four glasses of water to flush the liver.

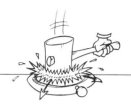

Time Stopper

Those potent little shots of wheatgrass juice—formerly almost exclusively consumed by "health food nuts"—are rapidly gaining in popularity. Rightfully so. They are power-packed with a rich variety of vitamins, minerals, and trace elements. In fact, it would take 25 pounds of vegetables to equal the nutritional power in one pound of fresh wheatgrass.

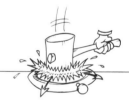

Time Stopper

Once upon a time, medical doctors pooh-poohed herbal remedies as "old wives' tales" and "snake-oil cures." Nowadays, thanks in part to best selling authors, Gary Null and Dr. Andrew Weil, Public Television, and National Public Radio, more and more physicians and medical schools are acknowledging the importance of herbs and nutrition in a total health care package.

This is just a sampling. We would have liked to have given you a complete list of every known herb, spice, and healing food, but we had to settle for tantalizing you into experimenting on your own. We hope we've succeeded.

You'll find these healing plants as roots, stems, seeds, leaves, and flowers, as well as in the form of powders, capsules, tablets, and teas.

Think of it as an adventure through nature's garden.

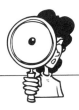

WatchWord

Aromatherapy uses the aromatic essential oils extracted from plants and flowers for both healing and cosmetic benefits. To be used safely, these volatile essences must be diluted in alcohol or nonessential oils.

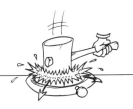

Time Stopper

Your favorite-smelling essential oils, when mixed with a high-quality cold-pressed carrier oil, such as almond, sesame, and grapeseed oils, make a great bath or all-over body oil.

Water's for More Than Thirst

Everyone knows that water is vital for life.

What you may not know is the enormous amount the body needs to carry out its vital functions. There is no single bodily function that doesn't need to be completely immersed in water.

Don't expect the instinct of thirst to indicate how much your body needs. Since the kidneys filter 4,000 to 8,000 quarts of blood daily, they need ample water to do this job effectively. Here're some more factoids about how much water the body uses every day:

➤ Two to three pints for each meal to be digested.

➤ Two to three pints for perspiration.

➤ Two to four quarts moisture exhaled by the lungs.

➤ Two to four quarts eliminated by the kidneys.

And, particularly interestingly, one to three pints per hour of flying time. The humidity aboard an aircraft is only 1 to 3 percent.

Let's drink to that ... water, that is!

Aromatherapy—Some Common Scents

Not too far removed from the study of healing foods is the art and science of *aromatherapy*. In fact, you'll notice that several commonly used essential oils are derived from food sources.

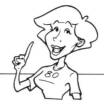

Voice of Experience

Asked to summarize the power of aromatherapy, Patricia Betty, director of The Aromatherapy Institute in New York City and author of *Aromatherapy: A Personal Journey Through the Senses* (Carnegie Press, 1994), replied eloquently, "Oils are unconditional liquid love."

Patricia Betty, master aromatherapist, explains that the controlled use of the aromatic essential oils present in plants deeply affects a person's physical, mental, and emotional state.

Beyond Smell

Aromatherapy embodies far more than scented soaps and candles. It is a highly developed fusion of art and science that goes far beyond our sense of smell. Essential oils reach us at three levels:

➤ Through touch, as diluted oils are applied to our skin

➤ Through inhalation, to the lungs

➤ As they cross through the body/brain barrier to affect our sense of well-being

It Makes Scents

Here's a sampler of essential oils commonly used in the practice of aromatherapy. It's refreshing to see how many are finding their way into health food stores and drugstores.

Be aware that the therapeutic properties listed for the following oils are not intended to be prescriptions for illness.

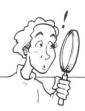

Age Alert

Caution: Aromatherapy oils are very potent and can be toxic in undiluted form. Certain commercial brands readily available at drugstores and department stores come premixed in safe proportions. Don't apply undiluted oils directly to the skin or take internally unless under the care of a reputable aromatherapist. You can safely use diluted oils for your bath or on your skin.

Essential Oil	Therapeutic Property
Anise	Digestive tonic Respiratory aid Headache relief
Basil	Nerve tonic and relaxant Antiseptic Decongestant Cough suppressant
Bay	Uplifter Decongestant Refresher Astringent
Bergamot	Antiseptic Antispasmodic Appetite stimulant Skincare Eczema Tanning
Birch	Cooling Cleansing Antiseptic Decongestant
Chamomile	Also known as azulene Appetite stimulant Fights dizziness and insomnia Calmative Treatment for burns, sunburn, sensitive skin
Camphor	Analgesic Antiseptic Diuretic Stimulates circulation, respiration, digestion Treats insect bites Sedative properties
Carrot	Skincare Rashes Antiwrinkle preparation Skin softener
Cedarwood	Calming Expectorant Antiseptic Acne treatment
Cinnamon	Antiseptic Stimulates digestion Relieves insect bites, stings Breath freshener Soothes toothache, gum pain

Essential Oil	Therapeutic Property
Citronella	Insect repellant
Cloves	General tonic Analgesic Antispasmodic Antiseptic Stops toothache pain Gum treatment Insect repellant
Coriander	Analgesic Antispasmodic Appetite tonic Relieves rheumatic pain
Cypress	Mood elevator Antispasmodic Muscle relaxant Pertussis
Eucalyptus	Decongestant Respiratory, circulatory stimulant Relieves joint pain Disinfectant Insect repellant
Fennel	Antiseptic Antispasmodic Bruising Digestive tonic Appetite stimulant Decongestant Gum treatment
Frankincense	Uplifting tonic Sensitive skin Expectorant
Garlic	General tonic Antiseptic Diuretic Digestive aid Carminative Parasiticide Vascular antispasmodic
Geranium	Circulation tonic Skin balm for dry skin, complexion Burn treatment
Ginger	Antiseptic Analgesic

continues

continued

Essential Oil	Therapeutic Property
	Warming
	Digestive tonic
	Muscle pains
Jasmine	Astringent
	Antispasmodic
	Treatment of acne
	Sensitive skin and wounds
	Muscle relaxant
Juniper	Acne
	Skincare
	Water retention
	Baths
Lavender	Mood elevator/calming
	Antiseptic
	Disinfectant
	Restorative tonic
	Coolant
	Bactericide
	Decongestant
	Intestinal stimulant
Lemon	Appetite stimulant
	Digestive tonic
	Circulatory stimulant
	Relieves insect bites, stings
Lemongrass	Stimulant
	Astringent
	Revitalize
	Digestive tonic
Marjoram	Calming
	Relieves anxiety, insomnia
	Expectorant
	Analgesic
	Fortifying baths
	Digestive tonic
	Respiratory tonic
Myrrh	Skin balm
	Antiwrinkle
	Sedative
	Warming
	Gums
Nutmeg	Analgesic
	Carminative
	Digestive tonic
	Toothache remedy

Essential Oil	Therapeutic Property
	Rheumatism Baths
Orange	Antiseptic Mood uplifter Skin balm Relaxant Heart tonic
Orange blossom (neroli)	Astringent Euphoric Nerve tonic Relieves cardiac spasms Skincare treatment
Patchouli	Uplifter Tonic Skincare Deodorant Perfume fixative
Pennyroyal	Analgesic Decongestant Insect bites, stings Bruises Itching **Caution: Pregnant women should never use this as it may induce contractions.**
Peppermint	Mood uplifter Carminative Antiseptic Analgesic Antispasmodic Breath freshener Decongestant
Pettigrain	Spicy orange-scented fresher Uplifter
Pine/Fir needle	Antiseptic Tonic Stimulant Treatment for rheumatism Used in baths
Rose	Astringent Carminative Sedative Skincare
Rosemary	General tonic Cardiotonic

continues

continued

Essential Oil	Therapeutic Property
	Carminative
	Decongestant
	Brain stimulant
	Breath tonic
	Antineuralgic
	Parasiticide
	Aphrodisiac
Rosewood	Spicy rose scent
	Mood elevator
	Skin balm
	Refreshing bath
Sage	General tonic
	Astringent
	Antispasmodic
	Calmative
	Antiseptic
	Decongestant
	Muscle relaxant in bath
Sandalwood	Circulatory stimulant
	Astringent
	Relaxant
	Tonic
	Aphrodisiac
Sassafras	Stimulant
	Astringent
	Relieves rheumatic pains
	General tonic
Spearmint	Digestive aid
	Decongestant
	Analgesic
	Parasiticide
	Antiseptic
	Breath freshener
	Deodorant
	Mood elevator
	General tonic
Tangerine	Antiseptic
	Gentle mood uplifter
	Skin tonic
	Relaxant
	Heart tonic
Tea tree	Antiseptic
	Antifungal
	Disinfectant

Essential Oil	Therapeutic Property
	Wounds treatment
Thyme	Antiseptic
	Bactericide
	Circulatory stimulant
	Expectorant
	Carminative
	Relieves hypertension
	Digestive, nerve tonic
	Parasiticide
Vetivert	Calmative/balancer
	Woodsy grass scent
Wintergreen	Strong camphoric mint
	Analgesic
	Digestive aid
	Decongestant
	Analgesic
	Antiseptic
	Breath freshener
	Mood elevator
	General tonic
Ylang-ylang	Sedative
	Calmative
	Relieves hypertension
	Regulates heartbeat

So ends our aromatherapy apothecary. Hattie's been having aromatherapy massages for more than 20 years and looks forward to enjoying at least another 20. If you haven't experienced one yet, give yourself a gift.

The Least You Need to Know

➤ Plants have been used medicinally for centuries.

➤ Everyday spices and herbs from the kitchen have healing properties.

➤ A new breed of physicians is beginning to incorporate the use of herbs into the practice of Western medicine.

➤ Drinking inadequate amounts of water causes premature aging.

➤ Aromatherapy uses concentrated essential oils that heal and uplift the body, mind, and spirit.

➤ Shopping for herbs, spices, and aromatherapy oils can be a fulfilling adventure in healthy living.

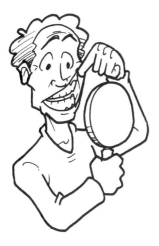

Chapter 24

Of Time, Teeth, and Cosmetic Surgery

In This Chapter

➤ Knowing how your face and body change with age

➤ Checking out the condition of your mouth

➤ Looking at laminates and other corrective dental procedures

➤ Erasing lines and wrinkles with acupuncture

➤ Considering plastic surgery

➤ Knowing what to expect from a face-lift

➤ Looking into body-contouring operations

An attractive, accomplished woman in her early 50s caught a reflection in a mirrored department store window and stopped transfixed. "I saw my mother walking right beside me," she laughed. "That is, I *thought* I saw her. Then I realized that the 'older' woman I'd spotted out of the corner of my eye wasn't mom, it was me."

She added, "My mother was a beautiful woman, but to me, she was always 25 years older than me. She was always, in a word, matronly. I feel neither old nor matronly."

Rather than dwelling on the fact that the face and body she sees in the mirror no longer match her mental self-portrait, she began to explore ways she could bring her body and spirit into alignment.

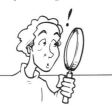

Age Alert

You aren't your body. Don't judge yourself solely by physical standards. Isn't it interesting that people who've always been considered attractive generally have a harder time dealing with aging than those who are of average looks? Seems they have more to lose!

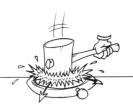

Time Stopper

Most mouthwash that kills germs contains alcohol. Since alcohol gets absorbed into the bloodstream, look for a mouthwash that contains no alcohol. You'll find brands in health food stores and many large drugstores.

The face you see in the mirror is not the face frozen in time in your high school yearbook. It's not even the face in your wedding pictures.

In this chapter, we'll discuss some of the options open to us to keep ourselves looking *physically* youthful. If you don't like what you see, you have plenty of options to consider, starting with a trip to your dentist to make sure your mouth is as young as possible.

Time's Toll on Teeth

As we did in Chapter 3, "What Does Your Mouth Say About You?" we're turning to Dr. Gerry Herman of New York's Park 56 Dental Group for advice on keeping teeth and gums in top condition.

Regrettably, time takes its toll on our smiles. Unlike in George Washington's day, when "choppers" were made of wood and toothless was the only other option, today's dentistry can restore and beautify even the most time-worn teeth. Prostheses—dentures, implants, and bridgework—look real, not like Chiclets, and even 50-year-olds are getting braces to correct imperfections they've lived with for years.

Your Dentist Really Can Make You Smile

New techniques that brighten and repair your teeth go a long way to restore a youthful smile. This can be as simple as whitening your teeth with a bleaching solution or as complex as orthodontia.

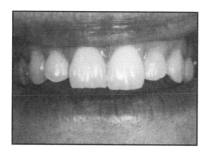
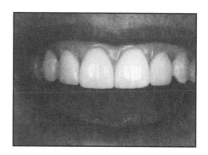

Skillful dentistry gave this patient something to smile about. The two front teeth and the two canines were slightly reshaped with a diamond burr, saving the patient a lot of unnecessary work. Porcelain laminates were then applied to the two teeth on either side of the front teeth.

(Photos courtesy of Dr. Gerry Herman)

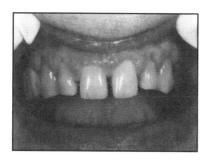
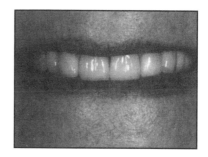

Dr. Gerry Herman applied porcelain laminates to close the gaps between this woman's six front teeth. With proper care, this will last for 10 to 15 years.

(Photos courtesy of Dr. Gerry Herman)

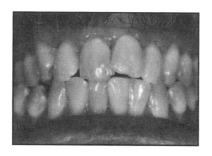
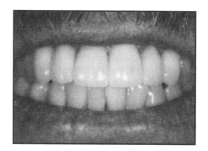

This patient's teeth were not just stained, they were chipped and crooked. First the teeth were bleached and then, after extensive preparation, the overlapping front teeth were laminated for an even, perfect shape. Other teeth were reshaped with a diamond burr to create a young-looking mouth.

(Photos courtesy of Dr. Gerry Herman)

Whiten and Brighten Your Smile

The simplest, most economical, and least-invasive way to brighten your teeth is bleaching. This involves treating the teeth with a peroxide-type solution and a light.

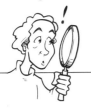

Bleaching takes several applications over a period of several weeks to lighten stains and discolorations.

Generally an office procedure, bleaching is usually done by one of the dentist's technicians.

Sometimes treatments begin in the office to jump-start the bleaching process and then continue at home. A tray is fitted to the teeth, and the patient is given a solution to be used at home for a couple of weeks.

Bleaching can be repeated as often as you want or need. It is safe enough to use often without damaging the enamel, dental work, and gums.

Some people experience sensitivity to cold drinks or ice cream during the time they are bleaching their teeth.

Age Alert

When choosing colors for dentures and laminates, don't pick one that is too light or too bright white. This won't make you look younger or more attractive. Your teeth will just look fake.

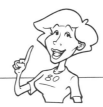

Voice of Experience

New York prosthodontist Dr. Gerry Herman advises, "If the shape and size of your teeth are fine but the color isn't, ask your dentist about bleaching. If the spaces between your teeth are wide, or you don't like the size and shape of your teeth, laminates can give you the teeth you've always wanted. Laminates can close spaces and even out your teeth."

Bonding/Laminates

Some flaws can be corrected by bonding wafer-thin porcelain veneers—laminates—to your less-than-perfect teeth. Custom-made by a lab so that they fit your teeth precisely, laminates are bonded onto your teeth to fill in spaces and even out the shapes.

Before porcelain laminates were invented, dentists tried to bond teeth with a plastic bonding material, filling in chips, for example, to make the tooth appear whole.

Dentists applied this composite resin material directly to the tooth and attempted to shape it as needed. It was difficult to produce good results, and the resin bonding material could stain and chip.

Lest you think dentists no longer use composite resin, those beautiful white fillings you got to replace your old silver fillings are all bonded.

Adult Orthodontia

Nobody has to have crooked teeth, regardless of age. As technology grows, more adults than ever are opting to wear braces to correct crowding, malocclusion, and misaligned bites.

Orthodontia is also used as a precursor to mouth restoration. Often teeth are extracted as a precursor to crownwork and bridgework. Orthodontic appliances can widen spaces so that a proper bridge can be made or laminates can be made to fit more easily.

When considering orthodontic treatments, explore different kinds. Some can even be put behind the teeth where they won't be visible. Also determine if the practitioner has plenty of experience in fitting braces on adults.

The time orthodontia takes varies, depending on the work needed. On the average, minor correction takes six to nine months; more extensive work takes a couple of years.

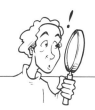

Age Alert

If you have silver fillings in your teeth, be aware that they contain a high percentage of mercury, which is highly toxic. Seek out a dentist experienced in safely removing mercury fillings and replacing them with nontoxic materials. You'll not only be saving your health, but these new, improved fillings are white and beautiful.

Dr. Herman's Ten Rules for a Youthful Mouth

Here are 10 rules to follow that will keep your mouth and teeth in the best possible condition:

1. Keep your lips moisturized.
2. Brush your teeth with the intention of cleaning every surface on every tooth. Use a soft-bristled toothbrush, and spend at least two minutes cleaning your teeth. If you wear any type of removable dental prosthesis, you need to keep it sparkling clean as well.

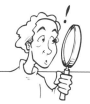

Age Alert

Laser treatments to lighten teeth are emerging as cutting-edge technology. Just make sure that your dentist is an expert in this process.

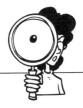

WatchWord

Orthodontia is the dental specialty concerned with correcting irregularities in the teeth by bringing the teeth into proper alignment. This is accomplished by using wires and bands to move the teeth into place.

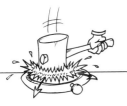

Time Stopper

You might not have to spend thousands and thousands of dollars on laminates. A dentist with a good eye and a deft hand can reshape teeth with a fine diamond burr.

3. Learn how to floss properly, and do it after every meal.

4. See your dentist for a professional cleaning and examination once every six months—more if you have a periodontal (gum) condition.

5. Have broken teeth restored, and have missing teeth replaced. Discolored and stained teeth can be bleached and otherwise whitened. Metallic fillings and restorations can be replaced with newer and safer aesthetic composite resins or porcelain restorations.

6. Take 1,000 milligrams of vitamin C per day to help keep gums healthy.

7. Drink lots and lots of purified water, and eat plenty of fresh fruits and vegetables. Reduce or completely eliminate refined sugar products from your diet.

8. Don't smoke cigarettes or use any type of tobacco—cigars, pipes, chewing tobacco. Don't drink excessive amounts of coffee or tea. The exception is herbal tea.

9. In front of a mirror, practice exaggerated mouth movements, such as smiling broadly, moving the lower jaw from side to side, and sticking your tongue out as far as you can. This helps to keep the muscles around the mouth toned and the jaw joints flexible.

10. Don't do anything with your mouth or teeth that might cause damage, such as opening envelopes, ripping tape, chewing on objects, biting your fingernails, etc. Wear a mouth guard when engaging in athletic activities. Have your dentist construct an occlusal guard for you if you clench or grind your teeth.

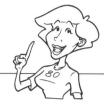

Voice of Experience

For shining teeth and healthy gums, mix a paste of baking soda, sea salt, and hydrogen peroxide and brush as you would with a drugstore paste. This from Hattie, who never uses toothpaste: "I've been using this recipe for more than 10 years, and my dental hygienist never fails to remark on the outstanding condition of my gums."

Getting a Lift from Acupuncture

If extraordinary skincare and the Lift Your Face exercises from Part 3 aren't keeping your face and neck as young-looking as you'd like, what are your options? Not everybody wants to rush into surgery just to smooth out a few wrinkles.

Acupuncture may be your answer.

"The results are dramatic. You can see them almost at once," explains Florence Patsy Roth, L.Ac. Despite rapid visible improvement, however, a course of 10 treatments is necessary to produce long-lasting results.

The acupuncturist places needles as fine as hair into fine lines to stimulate the circulation of blood and **lymph** throughout the face and head. This also can bring more contraction or tone to flaccid muscles in the cheeks and jowls as well as across the brow line.

Ms. Roth, whose practice is in New York's Greenwich Village, notes that there's another bonus to facial acupuncture: It clears your sinuses.

She adds, "Acupuncture is about an inner well-being that shows up in the face. You cannot work on the face without working on the whole body. Acupuncture does stimulate good, strong blood circulation through all the places that need blood, but this blood must be healthy. So we also work with people to change their diets so that their blood is as rich and nutritious as blood can be."

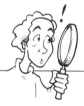

Age Alert

Aspirin, which is often taken to retard cardiovascular disease, has blood-thinning qualities that can contribute to bleeding. Your doctor and dentist also need to know if you use nicotine gum or patches in an effort to stop smoking. These seemingly mundane things could affect your course of treatment and recovery. Remember: Just because medications are over-the-counter does not make them harmless.

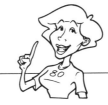

Voice of Experience

According to the American Society of Plastic and Reconstructive Surgeons, about 87 percent of all cosmetic surgery operations are performed on women.

Preparing for Plastic Surgery

Plastic surgery is not the solution for everyone who wants to look younger, but it does offer a wide array of options.

You might consider a chemical peel to smooth damaged skin on your face or to lighten age spots on your hands, or you might go for breast enlargement (or reduction), or liposuction to get rid of your love handles or saddlebags.

Just remember, when going for cosmetic surgery, less is often enough. Once a tummy is tucked or eyelids lifted, if the doctor removes too much tissue, you can't have it put back.

Whatever you think you want to do, do your research. Find out all the risks.

And make sure your expectations about the results match up with what the surgery can do.

Also, if money is an issue, be aware that most plastic surgery is considered elective and, as such, is rarely covered by insurance.

According to Dr. Richard A. Marfuggi, "If you want to have your breasts enlarged in order to be more comfortable about your body, that's fine. However, if your husband is pushing you to have this procedure to fulfill *his* fantasies, you might want to think a bit longer before scheduling an operation."

A board-certified plastic surgeon who has been practicing in New York City since 1982, Dr. Marfuggi adds, "With a healthy motive and realistic expectations, you will maximize your benefits and increase your chances for success and satisfaction."

Whatever operation you're considering, do your research. Shop around. Interview doctors and find out how many tummy tucks they do in a year—if that's what you're thinking about having. You do want your surgeon to have lots of experience in your operation, don't you?

Dr. Marfuggi, author of *Plastic Surgery: What You Need to Know Before, During and After* (Perigee), says "Obviously, finding the right plastic surgeon is more than checking in the Yellow Pages under 'Plastic Surgeons' or responding to an advertisement. You can't even tell how good or how reputable a doctor is by the address, fee schedules, media attention, or roster of celebrity clients."

Ask friends or anyone you know who's had a procedure like the one you're considering, your family doctor, nurses (operating room nurses are a great source), your community medical center, and the American Society of Plastic and Reconstructive Surgeons for referrals. Collect names, and ask for a consultation with three or four who are high on your list.

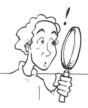

Age Alert

Pregnant women should *not* have anesthesia. The drugs used in surgery—even dentistry—and anesthesia can harm the fetus and cause birth defects. If there is any possibility that you might be pregnant, see your family physician or gynecologist to exclude this possibility *before* having any surgery or anesthesia.

The Least You Need to Know

➤ Your face and body keep changing as you age.

➤ For a great smile and youthful appearance, keep your teeth and gums in top condition.

➤ For realistic-looking dentures, bridgework, implants, and laminates, choose a color that *is* not too white.

➤ The simplest, most economical, and least-invasive way to brighten your smile is with bleaching.

➤ Porcelain veneers laminated to your teeth can fill spaces and give you perfect-looking teeth.

➤ Acupuncture can "lift" your face without surgery.

➤ Shop around for a board-certified, experienced plastic surgeon before committing to an operation.

Part 6

Living a Life You Love

We've been programmed to believe that aging goes only one way—downhill.

By the time you reach this part of the book, you'll have learned how you can reverse many of the less-desirable physical aspects of growing older by changing your approach to eating, exercise, and skincare. You'll also know that the right attitude goes a long way toward determining the course of your aging.

Mastery of the four E.A.S.E steps empowers you to create a life you love. Imagine what a relief it is to be free of the ravages of time. Instead of fearing aging, you can face it head-on with optimism and joy.

Imagine how great it would be to enjoy satisfying sex at every age, and how time has allowed you to develop an extraordinarily deep sense of self-worth. All this will allow you to design a life that satisfies you and inspires all those around you.

With this renewed self-confidence, you can proudly assert:

"I claim my life as an adventure, an opportunity, and a gift."

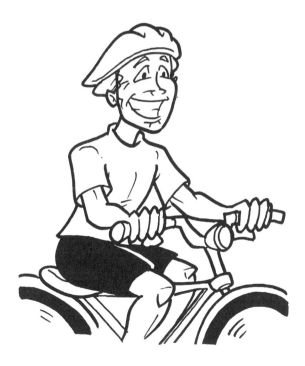

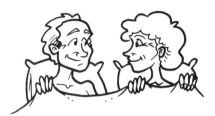

Chapter 25

Great Sex Has No Age

In This Chapter

➤ Sex when you were young

➤ What sabotages sexual pleasure

➤ Male dysfunction and menopause

➤ It's more than just intercourse

➤ Communication is key

Most sexual problems start much earlier than age 50, but after that, they just seem to escalate. Too many people accept this as normal and sit back waiting for the inevitable to happen. We totally disagree. We believe that waning sexuality is NOT a necessary part of aging.

We've been brainwashed to believe that our sex drive diminishes with age.

It doesn't have to.

We've been brainwashed to believe that we will become undesirable, impotent, even pathetic.

We don't have to.

We don't know exactly how—or why—these negative myths got started, but we do know that every one of them can be dispelled … and must be for us to truly enjoy a fulfilling sex life.

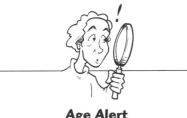

Age Alert

Our most important sex organ isn't our genitalia—it's our brain.

Different, but Still Great

Wouldn't it be a colossal waste if we became wiser and wiser with the passage of years, only to lose our sexuality? Sex at 50, or even 40, isn't exactly like it was in our 20s, but then neither is anything else. The trick is not to bemoan what *was* but to savor what *is*.

There is absolutely no reason for you to be deprived of your youthful passions—the ones you feared were going, or have gone, forever.

Great sex is everyone's birthright. The time has come for you to reclaim yours—starting now.

The Good Old Days When Sex Seemed Simple

How is it that, whatever the reality, we tend to recall our earliest sexual experiences as romantic, wild, and wonderful—a piece of cake?

And why is it that now that we're older, free to enjoy sex any time and place we want, sex that once was perceived as glorious shows up as troublesome, boring, and fraught with problems?

For some reason, no matter how mature and accomplished we are in other areas, we still approach sex using outdated standards based on our earliest experiences. Decisions we made decades ago still color our reactions and expectations, even though they no longer make sense and cause us considerable grief.

Something's definitely off here.

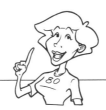

Voice of Experience

Hattie has heard similar complaints from countless clients. "I found that, whether they are aware of it or not, even highly successful, mature individuals approach sex with outdated expectations. When I suggest that they appreciate themselves as they are right now, they fight me. They refuse to accept the fact that a mature person can give and receive enormous sexual pleasure. Instead they opt to struggle to recapture their past prowess, competing with memories of their youth. This is sexual self-destruction."

And How Was It for You?

To get a sense of how you formulated your concepts of sex, think back to your earliest experiences. Do you remember how you felt? Were you frightened or exhilarated, or both? What conclusions did you draw? What about your partner? Did anyone make you feel guilty or ashamed?

As you continue to reflect on these early encounters, you will understand the origins of your current opinions and decisions. It's only after acknowledging how bound you have been to your past that you can release its hold on you.

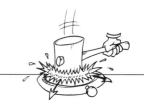

Time Stopper

Holding on to beliefs and behaviors from the past impedes satisfying sexuality in the present. Let go of these preconceptions and set new standards aligned with who you are now.

Myths and Misconceptions

Often we don't realize how powerfully external events and attitudes influence even our most intimate moments. We *think* we are acting from our deepest feelings when, in fact, every move we make is tempered by the opinions of others and what we see and hear in the media.

As much as we may deny it, we have unconsciously absorbed stifling standards from our parents, teachers, and society that control us every step of the way.

Let's confront the subtle yet insidious influence society has imprinted on us and how these prevailing attitudes distort our sexuality.

Who hasn't bought into the ideas and images spoon-fed to us in magazines and movies? What we have been left with is the opinion that whatever *we* have doesn't cut it. Therefore, we are left feeling dissatisfied and inadequate, fantasizing about what great sex really would be.

And What Do You Think?

Which of these preconceptions about what constitutes great sex match your ideas?

➤ What you're sure everyone else is getting

➤ What you remember you once had

➤ What you fantasize you could have with another woman/man ... or two ... or more

➤ What you can't get with your mate

➤ What famous people have

➤ What you'd get if you lost your beer belly or cellulite

➤ What you think you would have if you had a bigger, thicker, harder penis ... or bigger, rounder, prettier breasts

➤ Anything but what you're getting

➤ All of the above

Actually, it's none of the above.

It may be a challenge, but you've got to get rid of these negative internal conversations if you want to restore passion to your life.

Think about it. How many of these myths do you still allow to sabotage your sex life?

How to Stop Sexual Sabotage

The only way to effectively stop sabotaging your sex life is to flip all outdated ideas and unrealistic expectations—anything that doesn't please or satisfy you—into actions and concepts that turn you on.

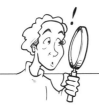

Age Alert

Stop putting pressure on yourself to have an orgasm—or several— every time you and your partner make love. Performance anxiety is certain to interfere with gratification. Quit counting orgasms. They are not the only measure of fulfillment. This also goes for erections.

There are four parts to this process:

1. The first calls for you to identify exactly what you believe to be true about sex that is diminishing your satisfaction.

2. The second is to get to the source—where, when, and from whom these unsupportive ideas originated.

3. Then, restate them in a form that reinforces your present needs and desires.

4. From this new perspective, take actions that provide gratification for who you are today.

This four-step process helps you escape the stranglehold your old ideas and behavior patterns have on your sex life.

Dealing with Male Dysfunction

All men have sexual anxieties from time to time, long before they reach middle age. The trouble is that they rarely talk about it, especially with their partners. They sulk in private, nursing feelings of inadequacy.

Thankfully, this may be changing as Viagra and other treatments for male impotence have found a voice on national TV. Nevertheless, a man experiencing sexual dysfunction often believes that he's the only one in the world to be inflicted so intensely. Secretly harboring such self-doubt only intensifies the problem.

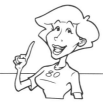

Voice of Experience

Before trying prescription drugs for male anxiety impotency, you might want to follow the suggestion of New York osteopath Dr. John Juhl. He recommends the amino acid L-Arginine as the safest agent for reducing this problem. The suggested dosage is 1,000 to 3,000 milligrams a day. This can be taken at one time or split into two doses. It increases circulation and helps blood vessels to dilate. The effect is felt in one hour. Look for it in your health food store.

Dealing with Doubts

A man who holds on to his youthful assumption that he can get an erection and sustain it for hours is setting himself up for disappointment when, in his mid 30s, this doesn't happen. The first time he might shrug it off because he's been working too hard or isn't really attracted to his partner. By the fifth or sixth time, he's convinced he's lost his manhood. After all, "real men" can get it up and keep it up whenever they want to.

This kind of thinking is dangerous.

Where did he get that idea? In the locker room after football practice when he was on the junior varsity squad in high school. Or from an older brother, or in the fraternity house, or plain old wishful thinking.

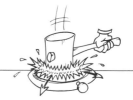

Time Stopper

It's a fable that what makes a man a passionate lover is that he can sustain a full erection for hours and hours. Holding on to this wildly unrealistic ideal robs many a man—and woman—of true sexual gratification.

Don't Fight It

You can see how you too might be tormented by such distorted expectations. The fact is that by the time they're 40, if not sooner, most men experience some degree of sexual dysfunction. Men who deny or fight this fact will undermine their ability to enjoy great sex.

Resistance keeps you from moving on to the next stage of lovemaking, which involves more foreplay and deeper intimacy with your partner. Yes, it may be different, but if you keep inventing new ways to give and receive satisfaction, you're on your way to enjoying the pleasures of mature sex.

While a man might not remain hard as often or for as long as he'd like, he can enjoy cuddling, kissing, fondling, stroking, and caressing for as many hours as he and his partner desire.

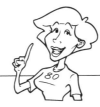

Voice of Experience

We want to share these touching quotes from a couple in their 80s who have been married for more than 60 years. Both recently underwent surgery for colon cancer and have found that their close brush with death has left them more in love than ever. The wife, 85, confided, "We've always enjoyed sex and now, even though we're older, and have both been seriously ill, our lovemaking has deepened. We cherish each other and our marriage is even stronger than ever." The husband, 87, spoke candidly, "Even though the physical aspects are more difficult, my desire is greater. It manifests itself in more touching and play, regardless of consummation. The pleasure and enjoyment is still quite great."

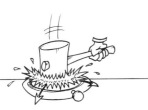

Time Stopper

For women during and after menopause, there are many safe, natural alternatives to hormone replacement therapy (HRT) that stop hot flashes, keep you lubricated, and restore diminished sexual desire. Consult your health care practitioner for support and advice.

Is There Sex After Menopause?

Men are not the only ones to be haunted by distorted sexual expectations. Many a woman has deprived herself of satisfying sex because she can't accept the changes in her body as she has matured. She may believe she is unattractive to her partner after she's had children or has begun menopause. She is convinced that time has stolen her beauty.

Hot flashes, cold sweats, and mood swings are just part of the picture. Women may have vaginal dryness, gain weight, sprout facial hair, and develop crêpe-like skin and age spots. Nobody has to suffer through these conditions. There are numerous ways to alleviate them, both medical and alternative. We talked about some of them in Part 5, "Dear Doctor," and you can explore other options with your health care practitioner.

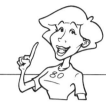

Voice of Experience

A 62-year-old widow confides that her sexuality remains so strong that she awakened in the middle of the night so aroused that, in her own words, "I was like a young boy having a wet dream. I wasn't even touching myself. Who would have thought I would still be so sexual at this age?"

Honoring Your Body

Discontent with the body is not only a function of aging. Think back to how critical you were about your body even when you were young. We women tend to obsess about every extra inch or pound. Even as young women, we turned off our partners with constant complaints about the size of our thighs, our stomachs, our breasts.

As mature women, we have had the opportunity to grow and deepen in character. Thankfully, we have gone beyond such petty concerns as an extra inch here or there. We have learned to appreciate and honor our bodies, despite their flaws. This is why so many older women are able to enjoy sex even more than when they were young. No longer impeded by fears of pregnancy and the discomfort of menstruation, we are free to fully enjoy open expressions of pleasure.

Playing Love Games

Coming from the point of view that everything and anything two lovers do with each other is okay as long as they both want it, let's explore innovative ways to give and receive sexual pleasure.

By now, you already know that there is more than one way to have sex. Intercourse is merely one of them.

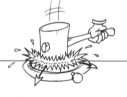

Time Stopper

For you men: In contrast to most men, a woman's enjoyment of sex can increase with age. When a woman has orgasms, her entire body quakes with the sheer pleasure of it. There's something happening to her that isn't happening to you. You can learn to have that, too ... and your mate can help you if only you learn to surrender. Relax and let your entire body enjoy the sensations. Don't be afraid to be passive. Enjoy experimenting with a side of you that might have been hidden.

275

Don't get us wrong: We're not putting intercourse down by any stretch of the imagination, but sexual pleasure entails far more than genital penetration.

There are all sorts of techniques for enjoying sex for the rest of your life. They do not focus exclusively on how well your genitals perform, but instead engage the *entire* body.

Get Creative

Create your own love games, starting with simply pleasuring each other's body with massage and lying together in the dark listening to music. You and your partner might find that you enjoy other less-traditional notions:

➤ Take a bath together—by candlelight or in the dark.

➤ Brush and comb each other's hair.

➤ Paint her toenails ... and ask her to massage your feet.

➤ Lick and kiss each other's toes, fingers, ears.

➤ Playfully bite, lick, pinch, scratch, tickle all over the place.

➤ Dance together naked in dim light or by candlelight.

➤ Do a seductive striptease.

➤ Practice *tantric sex*.

➤ Masturbate in front of each other.

➤ Look at sex magazines and videos together.

➤ Tie or blindfold each other.

➤ Invent role-playing games—here's your chance to play doctor again!

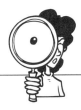

WatchWord

A style of making love that is Hindu in origin, **tantric sex** concentrates on the eroticism of the entire body. It requires that the male hold back from ejaculation for an extended period of time while the couple continues to pleasure each other without concentrating solely on the genitals.

The most exciting things can be ones that engage the unknown, what's forbidden, unexpected, or safely dangerous. Sex isn't only poetic and significant—it's also ridiculous and funny. So, play, play, play.

Let yourself be wild and weird. It's all judgment, anyway ... and you have to give that up to have great sex. People are ashamed of their pleasures, and shame sabotages sex.

It's More Than Just Intercourse

If you've ever listened in on a group of girlfriends dishing their husbands and lovers, or guys hanging out together, you've heard someone complain that sex has gotten boring and predictable, that it's lost its early excitement.

This goes right back to our original premise that we're hung up in our old stuff and keep expecting the same old formulas to take us to new heights.

Great sex doesn't work that way.

Relationships that become homogenized lose their spontaneity and excitement. They dry up.

You've got to keep inventing new ways to explore one another and release your old inhibitions. If time teaches us anything, it's to let go of the past. Sexual spontaneity can only flourish when we create each moment as it comes.

A good place to start is by admitting your hidden fantasies and desires, first to yourself and then to your partner. Invite each other to invent new love games that fulfill these fantasies. Here's a perfect opportunity to break free of those stifling judgments that can wreck a good relationship. What's more important, anyway?

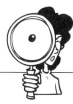

WatchWord

A **dominatrix** is a woman who works with clients, usually male, using bondage, discipline, and other expressions of sadism and masochism for sexual arousal and fantasy fulfillment. She may incorporate certain elements, such as psychodrama, role-playing, and control games.

Are Role-Playing and Domination for You?

One of New York's foremost *dominatrixes*, Mistress Carrie of the Arena Blaze Dungeon, reveals …

> We'd be out of business if women would accept and enjoy their lover's fetishes. Men come to us because we never make them feel ashamed for wanting to experience something that is too often considered unacceptable or even bizarre. For instance, society's standards say it's wrong, or weird, to practice S&M. We find that many perfectly healthy and well-adjusted men and women include this in their regular sex lives.
>
> The exchange of energy and trust is very important during any S&M play. Couples can start small with little games. I encourage them to write their fantasies down on pieces of paper, put them in a jar, then play a card game. The winner picks out one of the fantasies and then they play it out together. When both partners are on the same page, that's as good as it gets.

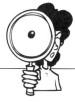

WatchWord

S&M refers to sexual practices involving sadism and masochism. This goes from simply tying each other up and using blindfolds all the way to spankings and other forms of punishment.

Fantasy Island

Fantasy games may be as simple as asking your partner to wear a sexy nightie instead of her usual ratty flannel granny gown, or as wild as asking if *you* can wear that same sexy nightie yourself.

Remember: Nothing that happens between two people who love each other is taboo if both partners want it. What keeps a relationship hot is this ongoing sexual exploration—without guilt, shame, or blame.

Your fantasies will keep changing. What turns you on will keep evolving as you and your lover develop increased trust and self-confidence. Inhibitions will just fall away, leaving great pleasure and play in their wake. What a gift.

Don't Lose It, Use It

Most people avoid talking about masturbation, despite the fact that they've done it for most of their lives. It is so rooted in shame that they feel guilty for feeling the pleasure it can provide. Some even refrain from masturbating as they get older.

This is unfortunate, since there is hard research showing that masturbation, like other sexual activity, stimulates the production of estrogen in women and testosterone in men. These hormones keep you looking and feeling younger. That in itself should encourage you to continue.

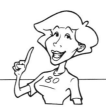

Voice of Experience

In his best-selling book, *Kosher Sex* (Doubleday, 1999), Rabbi Schmuley Boteach advises, "It follows that in lovemaking our ultimate objective is to transcend the body. We experience an intense pleasure that makes us feel really good about our partner, the object of our love. We have an out-of-body experience. We feel transported by the sexual encounter, lifted above the constraints of the body and meeting at the level of the soul. This is what orgasm is all about. It is an intensely unifying moment in which man and woman experience a spiritual epiphany."

Communication Says It All

Expressing your sexual fantasies isn't the only way you can enhance your relationship with your partner. After all, you don't spend all of your time in the bedroom.

And, like it or not, we often bring the stresses and resentments that irritate us in other areas of our lives to bed with us. This is hardly erotic, by anyone's standards.

Problems begin to emerge when we start to withhold criticisms of someone we love. After all, we don't want to upset them. Such withholding of truth, whether it is in word, deed, or emotion, stops love in its tracks.

Besides, who wants to walk around on eggshells? When you're concentrating on maintaining such a delicate balance, individuality and truth are lost. So what's the lesson in all of this? Both partners have to get real and stop being so darned sensitive. Stop obsessing over how your partner is going to respond if you don't act in a way you think he or she wants you to. Just be yourself, honestly and openly.

Be Childish

Take a lesson from kids. One says, "I hate you, poop-head. Go home!" whereupon the hated one picks up his or her toys and leaves. The next day, to no one's surprise, they play again. All is forgotten.

We don't advocate telling your beloved, "I hate you, poop-head. Go home!" We are, however, saying that you must add the element of play to your relationship. Lighten up. Encourage your lover not to get bent out of shape. And don't get bent out of shape yourself.

If you think about it, you'll get much further into a relationship with "poop-head" than someone you have reamed out with an epithet like "you controlling, insensitive bitch." Such personal assaults on another person's very being leave wounds that can take eons to heal, if at all.

When you have stopped communicating by shutting down completely and avoiding saying and doing anything to stir up controversy, an argument can erupt at any moment. You lose out on the joys of an open, fully expressed relationship.

Don't Be Thin-Skinned

Criticism doesn't have to hurt. You can actually learn to love it. Sounds strange. *Love* criticism? Yes, you can.

No kidding.

We tend to call anything we don't want to hear criticism. Then we don't have to pay any attention to it. On the contrary, we can learn a lot from these comments … especially those we particularly resist.

Learn to listen to what your lover tells you when it is expressed honestly, without malice or rage. You don't have to accept it, believe it, or act on it. Even though you may not agree with the content, the openness this kind of communication creates is liberating.

Stop being so thin-skinned and learn to forgive. As soon as you fully forgive someone for something they have said or done, the slate is cleared and neither of you is upset.

Train yourself not to make a production out of criticism. You can actually learn to love hearing people's opinions. They can be interesting. An insult can become a turn-on if you know it's coming from a place of honesty and care.

Ever notice how children playfully tease and jostle each other? This light-hearted interplay adds joy to their relationship and keeps it from getting heavy. Follow their lead.

Remember, it's impossible to have great sex when you're protecting your lover's feelings—or your own.

Let Down Your Guard

Truth is an astonishing aphrodisiac. Holding back is deadly. You will find that when revealing your hidden feelings becomes second nature, your sexual impulses will flow freely. You'll stop holding back. Your eroticism, excitement, and playfulness will reemerge with clarity and energy. You'll be interesting and adorable, like a child again.

We promise you that it's possible.

We promise you that it's worth it. Go for it.

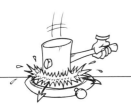

Time Stopper

Now that you've learned how sexually liberating open communication can be, you're ready to master the three Ls of successful sexual communication:

1. Listen
2. Lighten up
3. Laugh

The Least You Need to Know

➤ Early beliefs about sex influence us throughout our lives.

➤ Inhibitions sabotage pleasure.

➤ Enjoyment of sex changes as we age, not necessarily for the worse.

➤ There's more to great sex than just intercourse.

➤ Truthful communication leads to sexual satisfaction.

➤ Lighten up, listen, and laugh.

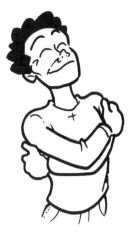

Chapter 26

Loving Yourself Through Time

In This Chapter

➤ Reversing the downside of aging?

➤ Facing your negative feelings about how you've aged

➤ Cultivating a sense of self-worth

➤ Hattietudes™ to lift your spirits

➤ Love is the answer

Is it possible to be 40, 50, 60, or even 90 and still feel vibrantly alive and productive? Yes, it certainly is.

History has provided us with inspiring role models—individuals who did not allow time to dull their appetites for life. Some who come to mind are Madam Curie, Georgia O'Keefe, Helen Hayes, George Burns, George Bernard Shaw, Rose Kennedy, Maurice Chevalier ... Regrettably, as you look about you, you can see too many discouraging examples of people who have aged poorly. We see the loss of vitality and waning spirit. This does not have to happen to you.

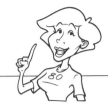

Voice of Experience

"The number of years one lives makes no difference. I say that there are no young and no old. Instead, there are two parts of life. The first is the working part, where one tries and works and tries to get ahead ... then comes the glorious second half of life, when like a river that starts as a rivulet, then cascades and then broadens into a great estuary ... the second half should start as early as possible. I was late, but what the hell! The second half, you do what you want. You have learned what you love to do. Now do it as hard as you can."

—Philip Johnson, 92, dean of American Architects, first director of architecture and design at New York's Museum of Modern Art, accepting an award at the Annual Aging in America Gala in 1999

Tarnish on the Golden Years

Nobody wants to be old and feeble. When people say they want to live a long life, they honestly do, just as long as they can remain active and alert. They are optimistic about the future, envisioning their "cruise ship years"—a golden time filled with all the travel they postponed while their careers and families were coming together.

We've never heard anyone say they want to live any longer than they are vital and in command of their bodies and their faculties. We certainly don't.

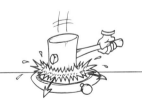

Time Stopper

Studies show that optimists live 19 percent longer than pessimists. Is your glass half full or half empty?

So What Goes Awry?

Much of the downside to aging can be attributed to neglect, abuse and misuse of the body. Those years of smoking, drinking, fatty foods, and sedentary evenings in front of the TV—instead of swinging a tennis racket or taking a walk—take their toll.

We chalk up aching joints and dimmed vision to part of the panoply of ailments generally regarded as *gerontological*. We become resigned to the failings of our bodies as inevitable and irreversible. That, coupled with a dreary view of the future, can make anyone's life dreadful at any age.

This is no way to honor and enjoy your life.

Attitude Affirmations Help You

Our mental images play a huge role in controlling how we age. If you expect to become incapacitated and incompetent, with wrinkled, sagging skin, it'll probably happen.

Can something be done about it? Yes. You can make the decision to turn it around.

One very effective way that we introduced in Chapter 13, "A = ATTITUDES That Keep You Young," is to use attitude affirmations. If you recall, these are powerful, positive comments to reverse society's negative views on aging that are imprinted on us in childhood. Once again, here they are:

➤ Acknowledge the negative thought.

➤ Then counter it immediately with an appropriate attitude affirmation.

➤ Finally, repeat this affirmation until the negative thought disappears.

This technique works for ideas, images, and thoughts about aging *in general*. But when you have to acknowledge feelings about your own aging, you have to delve much more deeply into yourself.

In this chapter, we ask you to face your *own* negative feelings about aging, not those of society.

We are emphasizing the negatives on purpose. This isn't to put a bad spin on growing older. Rather it is to get you to admit that you may be resisting and resenting aging with a vengeance.

Reversing your self-deprecating feelings can only happen through a deepening sense of self-worth.

That's the opportunity of aging.

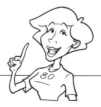

WatchWord

Gerontology is the scientific study of the aging process and the problems of aging people.

Voice of Experience

"The inner voice: the human compulsion when deeply distressed to seek healing counsel within ourselves, and the capacity within ourselves both to create this counsel and receive it."

—Alice Walker, novelist

Facing Your Negative Feelings About Aging

In this exercise, you will face your feelings about how you've aged. In the following table, write 10 aspects of your personal aging that you truly despise. Don't hesitate to say what's on your mind, no matter how brutal or unappealing it may be.

After finishing this list, write how each of these thoughts made you feel.

Undoubtedly, this will be very confronting. It was for us when we faced our own fears and self-doubts.

Facing Your Feelings

Part 1: 10 Ways I've Aged That I Hate:	Part 2: How This Makes Me Feel:
1. _____	1. _____
2. _____	2. _____
3. _____	3. _____
4. _____	4. _____
5. _____	5. _____
6. _____	6. _____
7. _____	7. _____
8. _____	8. _____
9. _____	9. _____
10. _____	10. _____

In this exercise, you uncovered your conditioned negative belief system around aging. You may even be amazed at how angry and even repulsed you are at the prospect of being old. It is only after you openly admit your fears, as you just did, that you will be able to counter this pervasive negativity.

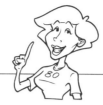

Voice of Experience

"Fear not, neither be discouraged."

—Deuteronomy 1:21

Isn't "Hate" a Bit Strong?

We decided not to avoid the word "hate," even though it is such a cruel emotion.

We believe that if you want to overcome anything (even hatred), you first need to recognize the part it plays in your life. Then if you want to release it, you can.

Denying that you have ugly, horrible thoughts only buries them deeper. Air them, share them— that's how you can break their hold on you.

As soon as you've acknowledged that you have all of these discouraging thoughts and feelings, you may feel temporarily trapped by this negativity. This won't last.

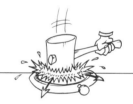

Time Stopper

Happiness is good for you. The hormones your body produces when you're happy keep you healthy, while those produced by sadness and stress break down the immune system.

Transforming your internal voice requires enormous focus and lots of mental effort. In fact, this is far more difficult than many physical challenges.

Your destructive messages about aging are deeply entrenched. They've been with you all of your life. We may have difficulty shaking free of them. Keep working at it.

Attitude Affirmations to the Rescue!

Here are some more attitude affirmations to help you through this process. They will empower you and strengthen your positive inner voice.

➤ I can't expect my feelings about aging to change overnight. They've been around for eons and hold on for dear life.

➤ I won't allow backslides to stop me. Backslides are absolutely to be expected. I'll keep affirming myself in the face of them.

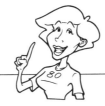

Voice of Experience

"Nothing in life is to be feared. It is only to be understood."

—Marie Curie

➤ I'll never be too old for really dramatic changes. Miracles happen at every stage of life.

➤ I'm ready, willing, and able to give up old concepts, habits, and possessions. Holding on to things from the past keeps me mired in it.

➤ Achieving a deep sense of self-worth allows me to value myself through whatever changes aging brings.

➤ I expect to get depressed, disgusted, and discouraged and will use my discontent as a springboard for transformation.

➤ Whenever I feel bad about myself, I'll call upon the concept of *creative self-disgust* to help me use my negativity as energy to make necessary life-affirming changes.

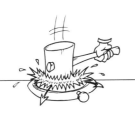

Time Stopper

Consider that what we think about aging is based on our past and the history of our Western civilization. It may be entirely off the mark and ready for major revision, culturally and personally.

Reprogramming Yourself— It Takes Work

Armed with your attitude affirmations, go back over the lists you made in your Facing Your Feelings exercise. Create powerful, self-affirming statements that override the depressing quality of your initial thoughts.

This will not be easy.

We are inundated with absolutely repulsive images—especially about ourselves—that keep cropping up no matter how hard we try to stifle them.

For example, if you wrote, "I hate that my breasts are drooping," and then, in the column where you acknowledged how this makes you feel, you wrote,

"I don't feel sexy anymore. No man will be attracted to me," you couldn't possibly feel any other way than awful.

The only way you can feel better about yourself after this crushing self-judgment is to create a meaningful, positive statement that reinforces your sense of self-worth. In response to our example, you might write, "I nursed both of my children with these wonderful breasts and am proud that my kids grew up healthy and happy. Moreover, I'm a beautiful woman—kind, loving, caring."

It takes constant work to provide ongoing antidotes to your habitually self-destructive inner voice. In time, you will be able to conquer it and replace it with warm, loving, encouraging attitude affirmations.

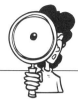

WatchWord

Creative self-disgust is a phrase we use to describe the use of constructive self-criticism as inspiration to make changes that move life forward.

Transforming Your Feelings About How You're Aging

For each of your statements and your corresponding feelings in the previous exercise, create an attitude affirmation to encourage a sense of self-worth:

1. _____
2. _____
3. _____
4. _____
5. _____
6. _____
7. _____
8. _____
9. _____
10. _____

Hattietudes

Hattie calls her favorite attitude affirmations Hattietudes. They give her an inspirational nudge to keep her spirits up when she's beset by self-doubt. She calls upon them to infuse her with renewed energy and a sense of self-worth.

In her private practice and lectures, Hattie encourages people to tack these Hattietudes onto the wall beside their desks, on their refrigerator doors, beside their bathroom mirrors—places where they can provide a lift throughout the day and for a lifetime.

In Chapter 13 we discussed the power of attitude affirmations to alter how we think about aging. Here are more of Hattie's favorite inspirational phrases:

➤ Never forget the YOU in YOUTH!

➤ Your first youth is a gift from Mother Nature; your second is a **gift** from yourself.

➤ Faith is the mortar of optimism.

➤ Optimism is the foundation of youth.

➤ Aging changes the "ME" Generation into *RE*generation.

➤ Age is never the reason, but often it's the excuse.

➤ Remember: IMPOSSIBLE = I'M POSSIBLE.

➤ The opposite of Old isn't Young, it's NEW.

➤ The path to youth is paved with possibility.

➤ Convert envy into inspiration, and you'll never run out of fuel.

➤ Age doesn't make you forget. It teaches you what's important to remember.

➤ Fighting Mother Nature is good exercise.

➤ Wrinkles don't make you old. Infants have plenty of them.

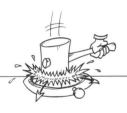

Time Stopper

Post your new image-boosting statements where you can see them—inside your daily planner, in your car where you can read them while stuck in traffic—and read them often. The best way to firmly plant them in your sub-conscious is to read them every night before you go to bed and again when you first awake in the morning. Self-hatred is tenacious.

➤ Never give up your dreams. They keep you awake.

➤ Beauty is never just skin deep.

➤ Don't let gravity get you down.

➤ Keep climbing and you'll never be over the hill.

➤ When life gets harder, you get smarter.

➤ The hands of time belong to you. Take aging into your own hands.

➤ Love is contagious. Go out and start an epidemic.

➤ Self-hatred doesn't come naturally; it's an acquired taste.

➤ Both blame and shame maim.

➤ Suffering is an option you don't have to pick up.

➤ If you were sexy when you were young, you'll be even sexier when you're older.

➤ Youth isn't wasted on the young—or on anyone else!

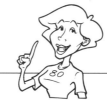

Voice of Experience

"All my life I have tried to pluck a thistle and plant a flower wherever the flower would grow in thought and mind."

—Abraham Lincoln

Loving Yourself Back to Youth

As The Beatles' tune goes, "All you need is love …"

We're in the midst of an epidemic of self-hatred, with aging as a prime target of this malice. Destructive images of aging that start in childhood erode our self-love.

One of the often overlooked blessings of aging is that it gives you time to learn to appreciate yourself, to develop a deep self-respect for who you have become.

Rather than focusing on every wrinkle or gray hair, learn to honor and love the person you are.

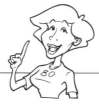

Voice of Experience

Says Hattie in her lectures, "When I first started transforming my negativity, there were many occasions when I lapsed into that old mode of thinking. But as hard as this process is, I decided that, no matter what my mind or society's unsupportive stance brought up, I would stay focused and grow younger with each passing year.

"Yes, I said grow younger. This may sound absurd. I certainly agree that it's an unusual statement, but I've made up my mind to marshal all my resources and transform aging, not only for myself and my clients, but for everyone else in the world who finds this prospect appealing."

Each of us is, in our own way, special. No one has lived life perfectly, but we've all brought our unique style of love, laughter, and joy to the world. With aging, it's especially important to remember how much we've contributed to those around us.

Do you recall that Christmas classic movie *It's a Wonderful Life?* James Stewart felt he was such a failure that he was ready to jump off a bridge and end it all. Once his angel Clarence showed how deprived the world would be had he never lived, he realized that he was loved, even if he couldn't love himself at that moment.

How often do we feel unworthy of love? Probably too often.

It is said that, with aging, comes wisdom. The wisdom that has the most enduring value, we believe, is the knowledge that each of us, individually, is remarkable.

Therein lies true self-love.

The Least You Need to Know

➤ You can change your pessimistic views about aging into life-affirming ones.

➤ Honestly facing your fears and discontents helps dispel them.

➤ A sense of self-worth is the antidote to negative thought and feeling patterns.

➤ Hattietudes give your attitude a boost.

➤ Love is, and always has been, the answer.

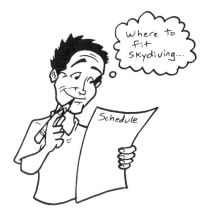

Chapter 27

Charting Your Future Youth

In This Chapter

➤ Fulfilling your dreams

➤ Happiness—the possible dream

➤ One last Blitz

➤ Being free and having fun

➤ Creating a style of life that suits you

➤ Transcending time

Here you are, at the last chapter, ready to design a future filled with joy and gratification.

When you were young, you always looked ahead. "When I grow up ..." is the phrase on every child's lips. And what about now, after you've grown up and achieved many of your dreams?

The answer is: Create new dreams.

What Lies Ahead?

For a future filled with youth, you'll begin by tapping into your deepest feelings—and needs—to live a life you love.

We're not suggesting that you build castles in the air and then try to move into them, but to create dreams that excite and delight you, then to take actions to make them come true. And, most of all, have faith and patience.

Hattie's Dream Future

In her book *RetroAge*, Hattie shares some of her dreams to inspire readers to let their fantasies soar. Here they are as she listed them in 1996:

➤ I will open five international RetroAge spas by the year 2001, the first on an island in the Caribbean. One of my tropical spas will be devoted to healthy families. I envision babies birthed in clear, warm water and mothers and fathers receiving exquisite care, along with their newborns. Furthermore, each spa will support local organic farming, humane treatment of animals, and clean water and air.

➤ I'll appear in an unretouched nude spread in *Playboy*.

➤ I'll star in a singing-dancing-comedy celebration of life at Radio City Music Hall.

➤ I'll host *Saturday Night Live*.

➤ I'll see the word "RetroAge" become part of the English language.

➤ My anti-aging chair design will be incorporated into offices, cars, and airlines.

➤ I even let my mind conjure up a satellite spa in outer space. The SpaShip RetroAge.

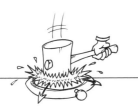

Time Stopper

Follow the lead of Anne Frank, who wrote in her diary, "Whoever is happy will make others happy too. He who has courage and faith will never perish in misery!"

Far-Fetched?

Granted, Hattie's dreams may seem wildly far-fetched, but she listed them, published them, and has set out to make as many come true as she can.

She hasn't played Radio City yet, but she did produce the Roseland Ballroom's 1999 Over-50 Bathing Suit Beauty Contest, handing over the title she had won 11 years earlier.

She also submitted unretouched photos to *Playboy*. While they declined her suggestion that they do a feature on the beauty of older women, the editor did say, "You certainly must enjoy a varied and exciting lifestyle. Best wishes to you as you continue to pursue your ambitions. Your vitality and enthusiasm are an inspiration to all of us!"

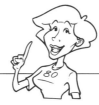

Voice of Experience

"I think the only reason you should retire is if you can find something you enjoy more than what you're doing now."

—George Burns

Let Your Fantasies Soar

We believe that working to make your dreams come true creates youth at any age.

We invite you to let your fantasies soar. Perhaps you won't reach *all* your goals—Hattie certainly hasn't yet—and perhaps you never will.

It really doesn't matter.

The power is in the act of creating dreams. They keep you awake, energized, and above all, young and exciting.

What Are Your Dreams?

Here's a written exercise called "Fulfilling My Dreams." In this, you will identify what you want from life. You will take dreams that have been floating around in your head—some for as long as you can remember—and write them down as specifically as you would the agenda for a business meeting. When doing this exercise, make sure to use words that inspire and empower you to take action—for in action lies ultimate fulfillment.

Don't worry if it they seem impossible. Keep focusing on them. Visualize and sense these goals until you can savor how it feels to be living them. Make your statements positive and powerful, even if your head keeps telling you "This can never be." We already know how discouraging our negative inner voice can be. Flip it with an attitude affirmation and go on.

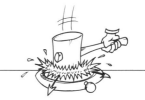

Time Stopper

Victor Hugo was on the right track when he wrote, "The supreme happiness of life is the conviction that we are loved."

Fulfilling My Dreams

Remember: Do not allow your inner voice, with its resignation and cynicism, to discourage you. No fantasy is taboo. Don't edit your thoughts. Follow your deepest, most inspiring fantasies rather than succumb to thoughts that tell you they're impossible to achieve. Give your imagination free rein as you do this two-part exercise.

Note: Don't be limited by the number of lines on these charts. Write down as many ideas as you can think of.

Part 1: What I've Always Dreamed of Doing

1. _____
2. _____
3. _____
4. _____
5. _____
6. _____

Part 2: What I've Always Dreamed of Having

1. _____
2. _____
3. _____
4. _____
5. _____
6. _____

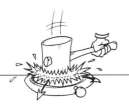

Time Stopper

Be inspired by this old Native American saying: "When you were born, you cried and the world rejoiced. Live your life in such a manner that when you die, the world cries and you rejoice.

Guilt-Free Desires

The joy in spinning dreams is that they have no limits. You can say, do, be, feel anything you want. After all, they're *your* dreams and desires. Don't fret over whether or not they will ever happen. And never, ever feel guilty for having them.

Stay in the moment and treasure the process.

We urge you not to be concerned even if you don't achieve any of your desires. Life is filled with surprises. Be open for the unexpected to happen, and something even better may come your way. You may have heard the expression "Life happens when you're doing something else."

What's important is that you do *something.*

Woody Allen is often quoted as saying "Just show up." And an athletic shoe company tells us "Just do it."

Perhaps you've held back from pursuing a life you love because you're afraid you'll fail. The only failure is in not trying at all.

Go for it.

You're in Good Company

As you open yourself to pursuing new adventures and fulfilling your dreams, you will meet more and more people who have made the same decision. They will welcome you and even help you, and you, in turn, will welcome and help others.

As psychologist Dr. John Kildahl says, "… It is extremely important that people who are growing older appreciate the importance of family, friends, and contacts with people. Networking becomes more and more important in terms of physical needs, but also in terms of emotional stimulation and inspiration."

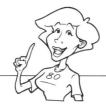

Voice of Experience

Radio and TV legend Joe Franklin hosted the longest-running TV talk show in history from 1950 to 1993. Now, at 71, he will be embarking on a new national TV venture, *The New Joe Franklin Show.* Speaking about his own longevity and spirit, with his "medical sidekick" Jonathan Silver, Ph.D., Mr. Franklin says, "There is a great deal of clinical research establishing the fact that there is a powerful medical value derived from our emotional power. In other words, aging is improved by a positive attitude, which helps you soar to higher altitudes. Keep the mind young, and the body will follow."

Two Who Pursued Their Dreams

We spoke with two individuals whose stories we believe are truly inspiring.

The first, Dr. Viana Muller, founded an international herb-importing company in her 50s. This achievement not only transformed her life, but it also allowed her to make an enormous contribution to humanity.

Second is former Golden Gloves winner Lou Bartfield. At the age of 62, he decided to return to the professional boxing ring and sued the boxing commission for age discrimination when it blocked his entry.

Here's what they have to say.

Viana Muller, Ph.D.

I found myself ill and out of work at age 50. I had finished my Ph.D. late—at 48—in anthropology. I wanted to get out and do something that would use my creative juices and would be of real benefit to people.

Being sick gave me time to read and research alternative medicine. During my recovery, I went to Peru with a friend to explore medicinal herbs.

The one herb that most excited us was maca, which we decided to import. Bringing this herb to America allowed us to revolutionize the way women handled menopause in the U.S. and other parts of the developed world where dangerous hormone replacement therapy had become very popular.

I had a double mission: to help American women—including myself—who were going through menopause and to help impoverished Peruvian communities by buying their maca roots at above-market value.

My associate, Elena Rojas, and I created Whole World Botanicals to fulfill this mission.

Founding Whole World Botanicals has given me the scope to create something a little out of the ordinary—a company with a social mission in addition to its dedication to being profitable. It stretches me beyond what I had ever imagined. It challenges me every day to have enormous faith.

Lou Bartfield

I went back into the ring at the age of 62. Because I was involved with vitamins, almost before everyone else, I stayed in condition for over 38 years. I didn't abuse my body with smoking and drinking, and worked out with boxers more than 30 years younger than me. That's why I felt ready to go back and box professionally again.

What I want to share with others is that the will of the human being, how we feel about ourselves, and what we think about ourselves is the important thing. You can have your ups and downs, just don't get stuck in them.

Think of yourself as very special and very unique. God gave you a gift … made you special. You have to use it. You have to practice and do whatever you have to do in a healthy, normal way that works over a life span.

What It Takes to Be Happy

It's easy to be lonely, discouraged, and depressed. With all that's going on in the world—and all our pressures to be a certain way or do certain things—these dismal feelings just show up uninvited.

Certainly, if you are beset by physical problems, or under constant financial pressure, or in a job you despise, you will have waves of sadness. You may even experience deep fear or depression.

Does this mean you can never be happy?

Of course it doesn't.

It means you're human, subject to the risings and fallings in life. The answer lies not in how often you fall, but how courageously you rise.

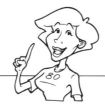

Voice of Experience

"If God told you exactly what it was you were to do, you would be happy doing it no matter what it was. What you're doing is what God wants you to do. Be happy."

—Werner Erhard, creator of the est Training, an intensely probing personal development program that positively impacted countless lives

Happiness has nothing to do with what you do or how much you have. It's a way of being that emanates from within, regardless of circumstances.

Every living soul has times of sadness, loss, fear, anguish, or pain. Of course, when we're caught up in the swirl of things, we can feel like we're alone in our anguish.

Regardless of what you see on TV, no one feels happy all the time. What we have to remember is that no one is exempt from problems. Therein lies our common humanity.

When we connect to the common bond of the human condition, we have the opportunity to feel compassion. Compassion is very close to love, and love is very close to happiness.

Love makes miracles happen.

Happiness is a miracle we all share.

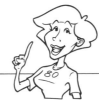

Clearing a Path for Your Future

You guessed it: another Blitz.

You Blitzed your kitchen to eat for youth and cleared your closets of clothing that's no longer flattering. You emptied cabinets of medicines and makeup that were accumulating and cluttering your life.

You won't be needing giant garbage bags this time. There's no physical clutter to handle. This Blitz involves clearing out …

- ➤ Memories.
- ➤ Ideas.
- ➤ Judgments.
- ➤ Expectations.
- ➤ Opinions.
- ➤ Relationships.
- ➤ Whatever is holding you back.
- ➤ Whatever is keeping you stuck in the past.

This final Blitz is not as tangible as filling giant garbage bags with things to throw or give away, but its effect on your life is every bit as powerful. Get ready to experience some deep feelings as you release these emotionally charged pieces of your past.

You'll Have to Take Risks

Just as children outgrow their clothing and toys, you outgrow things, too. When you ask yourself to take a hard look at whatever no longer serves you, you must be ready to give things up. This includes things you may have become very attached to, like where you live, or your career.

You may hesitate to make these changes for fear of being judged harshly or appearing irresponsible, impulsive, or selfish.

You may also be terrified that you'll be left without resources if you release too much.

Sometimes that's the chance you have to take to transform your life.

A Surprising Outcome to Sallie's Story

Sallie was elected to chair the board of an organization she had been associated with for years. This happened almost simultaneously with a big assignment that would really boost her career.

"After presiding over only three meetings, I found myself resenting the people I was close to who were part of the group. I resisted going to meetings. I had agreed to hold this position for a year and knew that my friends in the organization depended on me to represent them on the board. I was sure they would judge me harshly if I resigned. "I resigned anyway. Had I stayed on I wouldn't have been able to do *either* job effectively," she recalls. "My fears about resentment had been exaggerated. Strangers congratulated me on my promotion at work, and my friends, rather than being critical, were supportive. And I never felt freer."

All of Sallie's fears were in her head.

What Are You Afraid to Release?

Sometimes there won't be a happy ending. People may be upset and angry with you for sticking to your guns and taking care of yourself. That's their problem, not yours.

Look into your surroundings, your choices, your feelings. Check to determine if you are trapped in a way of being that is holding you back. Cultivate the courage to acknowledge what you must do, then do it.

Does this sound harsh? We think not. It can be absolutely liberating.

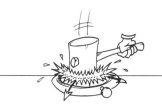

Time Stopper

To paraphrase an old adage, "He is happy who is happy with his lot ... or his little."

Creating a Life That Suits You

When we downsize our lives, clearing away "stuff" (both physical and emotional), we give ourselves room to explore possibilities we never even considered before.

Look at this as a playroom for your inner child. Arrange your life so that it is filled with everything, and everyone, you love. Then set your course toward only those things that serve you, that fulfill your dreams.

Have Fun!

We're serious about this: Aim to make everything you do fun. Children love fun. So do we all. Learn to let go of your stressful thoughts and feelings and play like a child.

This is not irresponsible, impractical, or frivolous. It provides you with a source of energy and inspiration that moves your spirit to stay young, regardless of your calendar age.

Life will be more joyous, and you'll be an inspiration to everyone around you.

Express Yourself Freely

One of the most enchanting characteristics of children is their candor. As we age, we socialize and, of necessity, learn to curtail the expression of our feelings. Did you ever hear a parent say, "Big girls don't do that," or "You're too grown up to cry?" We learn to refrain from saying what we see, think, and feel, lest we hurt someone's feelings or cause embarrassment. These withheld sentiments hold us back and make us inflexible.

The more you hold back, the older you get.

Free and open expression is one of life's greatest joys. With it, everything lightens up.

When you give yourself permission to openly express truth, the natural affection behind anger, fear, and judgment bubbles up, leaving a wake of intimacy and love.

What Are You Doing the Rest of Your Life?

Once upon a time, people worked at their profession for many years and retired in their 60s. Times have changed. Some people choose to retire in their 40s; some decide they'll work forever.

For some, after working for many years, retirement is a pleasing option. They plan to travel, attend concerts, dine out. They look forward to spending their time on hobbies and taking up activities they had no time for when they were on the job.

Others who can't imagine enjoying so much "leisure time" are drawn to a life of service. They envision themselves with a mission of making a difference.

There is no "correct" choice. Each of us has a personal destiny to pursue. Keep searching for yours and live life as fully as you can. Trust that there is a logic to the universe, and surrender to the beauty and bounty of life.

Transcending Time

You may not have the same skin or muscle tone you once had, but don't let that stop you from growing younger each day. True youth is vibrancy, energy, courage, joyfulness, and openness. And we never lose our God-given ability to generate these qualities for ourselves.

When this shift happens on the inside, your transformation will show on the outside. You will become ageless. Your stamina will soar. You will become stronger, more creative, courageous. You will lose the heavy burdens of worry and fear and experience a lightness of spirit. And, as a welcome consequence, you will look and feel younger.

Ageless

It is for us
Whom they call old
To stretch the borders of time
Across a silken sky
And to feel the yet-to-be
Brimming with flames and flowers
We dare not count the hours.

—Hattie

The Least You Need to Know

➤ Reawakening your dreams gives purpose to your future.

➤ Happiness comes from compassion and love.

➤ When you release whatever is holding you back, new possibilities emerge.

➤ You can retire or work forever, depending on what makes you happy.

➤ For some people, making a difference gives meaning to life.

➤ To transcend time, you must tap into your inner spirit.

➤ Spirit is ageless.

Forces and Sources

Here are some of our favorite sources of information and products. We've gathered them over the years and rely on their integrity and effectiveness to support our own RetroAging.

Web Pages and Other Resources

www.GenerationA.com

This well-written Web site is aimed at Americans who are 50 and older. There's news, plus features, interviews, and surveys.

www.ars-grin.gov/~ngrlsb/

This extensive database offers information about phytonutrients. It was assembled by Stephen M. Beckstrom and James A. Duke at the National Germplasm Resources Laboratory, Agriculture Research Service, United States Department of Agriculture.

www.ahealthylifechoice.com

April Okin's complete line of innovative products for a healthy life.

Aerobic Life
1-800-798-0707

An assortment of high-quality health products, including natural progesterone cream and aloe-vera juice.

Age In Reverse (AIR)
1-888-AGE-EASY

Antigravity Bodylift; fold-up foam and inflatable body slants for home use.

BD Herbs
1-800-760-3739

Herbal extracts, Demeter-certified Biodynamic organic herbs.

Belgravia Imports
1-800-848-1127

Sole U.S. Importers of Green & Blacks 100 percent organic chocolates, with 70 percent organic cocoa solids.

Biotec Foods
1-800-788-1084

Antioxidants, green papaya, sea plankton, digestive enzymes, soy isoflavons, cholesterol-lowering nutritional supplement; also nutritional products for animals (Hattie's favorites).

Bronson's Pharmaceuticals
1-800-235-3200

High-quality, reasonably priced pharmaceutical compounds. Ask for a list of natural products.

Diamond Organics
1-888-ORGANIC

Mail-order organic food catalog. Great gift packages.

E-Scentially Yours
212-545-0229
Fax: 212-545-1335

High-quality pure essential oils and blends.

Norwalk Juicer
1-800-643-8645

The Rolls Royce of juice machines—very expensive, with amazing extraction power.

Ocean Produce International
1-800-565-8773

Mineral-rich sea parsley, available dried and fresh.

Omega Nutrition
1-800-661-3529

Outstanding source of organic flaxseed oils, essential fatty acid (EFA) oil blends, cold-pressed culinary oils, fructo-oligosaccharides (FOS) prebiotic, coconut oil, saw palmetto, and stevia.

Pure Body Institute
1-800-952-7873

Liver, colon, and parasite herbal cleanse compounds made with more than 30 herbs.

Synergistic Health Concepts
1-800-594-4149

Methyl Sulfonyl Methane (MSM), Michrohydrin, and other nutritional supplements and skincare products.

Vegetarian Center of New York City
The Viva Vegie Society

212-414-9100

www.vivavegit.org

Publishers of *The Viva Vine*, a richly informative bimonthly magazine, and pamphlet, *101 Reasons Why I'm a Vegetarian*, by Pam Rice; consumer activists for animal rights.

Whole World Botanicals
1-888-757-6026 and 1-212-781-6026

Rain forest herbs, organic royal maca, camu-camu, chanka piedra.

Women's International Pharmacy
1-800-279-5708

Soy and Mexican wild yam hormone replacement therapy products; by prescription only. Human Growth Hormone (HGH) information only, 1-800-699-8143.

To order signed copies of *RetroAge: The Four-Step Program to Reverse the Aging Process,* call 1-212-388-8509 or e-mail RetroAge@aol.com.

Hattie is available for keynotes, workshops, seminars, TV, and newspaper and radio interviews. Contact 1-212-388-8509 or e-mail RetroAge@aol.com.

Bibliography

Balch, James F., M.D., and Phyllis A. Balch, C.N.C. *Prescription for Nutritional Healing, Second Edition.* Avery Publishing Group, 1997.

Betty, Patricia. *Aromatherapy: A Personal Journey Through Your Senses.* Carnegie Press, 1994.

——. *Essential Beauty.* Lowell House, 2000.

Brown, Susan E., Ph.D., *Better Bones, Better Body.* Keats Publishing, 1996.

Chopra, Deepak, M.D. *Ageless Body, Timeless Mind.* Three Rivers Press, 1993.

Clark, Hulda Regehr, Ph.D., N.D. *The Cure for All Cancers.* New Century Press, 1993.

Erhet, Arnold, *The Mucusless Diet Healing System,* Benedict Lust Publications, Inc., 1976.

Hattie, with Sallie Batson. *RetroAge®: The Four-Step Program to Reverse the Aging Process.* Berkley Publishing Group, 1997.

Hofstein, Riquette, with Sallie Batson. *Riquette's Grow Hair in 12 Weeks.* Harmony Books, Crown Paperback, 1988.

Kildahl, Dr. John, and Dr. Joseph Martorano. *Beyond Negative Thinking.* Plenum Publishing, 1989.

Lee, Helen. *The Tao of Beauty: Chinese Herbal Secrets to Feeling Good and Looking Great.* Broadway Books, 1999.

Lee, John R., M.D., with Virginia Hopkins. *What Your Doctor May Not Tell You About Menopause: The Breakthrough Book on Natural Progesterone.* Warner Books, 1996.

Magaziner, Dr. Allan. *The Complete Idiot's Guide to Living Longer and Healthier.* Alpha Books, 1998.

Marcus, Erik. *Vegan: The New Ethics of Eating.* McBooks Press, 1998.

Marfuggi, Richard A., M.D. *Plastic Surgery, What You Need to Know Before, During and After.* Perigee Books, 1998.

Null, Gary, Ph.D. *Gary Null's Ultimate Anti-Aging Program.* Kensington, 1999.

Ornish, Dean, M.D. *Everyday Cooking with Dr. Dean Ornish: 150 Easy, Low-Fat, High Flavor Recipes.* HarperCollins, 1996.

Robbins, John. *Diet for a New America.* Stillpoint Publishing, 1987.

Rosenfeld, Isadore, M.D. *Live Now, Age Longer: Proven Ways to Slow Down the Clock.* Warner Books, 1999.

Ryback, Dr. David. *Look 10 Years Younger, Live 10 Years Longer—A Woman's Guide.* Prentice Hall, 1999.

Sellman, Sherrill. *Hormone Heresy: What Women MUST Know About Their Hormones.* GetWell International, 1998.

Shippen, Eugene, M.D., and William Fryer. *The Testosterone Syndrome: The Critical Factor for Energy, Health & Sexuality, Reversing Male Menopause.* M. Evans and Company, 1998.

Walker, Dr. N.W. *Become Younger.* Norwalk Press, 1949. (still in print; see Appendix A, "Forces and Sources")

Glossary

aerobic Refers to heart function. Aerobic exercise is exercise that gets your heart pumping through repeated contractions of large muscle groups against low resistance. Walking, bike riding, playing tennis or basketball, dancing, cross-country skiing, jumping rope … all of these activities tend to burn lots of calories and, when done consistently and for a long enough time, contribute to weight loss.

allopathic (allopathy) Mainstream Western doctors routinely fight disease by relying on technology that focuses on the physical body, generally excluding the effects of the mind, body, and spirit.

alopecia An overall term referring to hair loss or balding. *Androgenic alopecia* is a hereditary condition evidenced by a receding hairline (male pattern baldness) or overall thinning.

antioxidants One of the best ways to combat free-radical damage is to consume plenty of *antioxidants*. This includes foods and supplements that are high in vitamins C and E and beta-carotene. Antioxidants also keep the formation of new free radicals in check.

aromatherapy Uses the aromatic essential oils extracted from plants and flowers for both healing and cosmetic benefits. To be used safely, these volatile essences must be diluted in alcohol or nonessential oils. Though they are not soluble in water, they will impart their scent if used in a bath. Aromatherapy oils are commonly used in fragrant bath and skin oils and scented candles.

arthritis The stiffening and inflammation of joints is the second-largest health problem to older people, second only to hearing loss. By age 30 (yes, that young), 35 percent of the population is plagued by osteoarthritis.

attitude affirmations Powerful, positive statements we say to ourselves to shatter the belief that we are no longer vital. These affirmations help silence the destructive inner voice that erodes our self-esteem as we age.

BEDCERCISES™ Highly effective stress-free exercises that are done in bed. When done in the morning before arising and again at bedtime, they increase flexibility of the joints and muscles.

Blitz The all-out elimination of anything that clutters our bodies, our minds, our spirits, and our homes. A Blitz clears away the past and prepares us for a youth-filled future.

BodyCheck   The act of facing different aspects of our bodies as they alter through the process of reversing aging.

chi   *See* qi.

creative self-disgust   A term we use to describe the use of self-criticism to inspire you to make changes that move your life forward.

detoxification   The thorough cleansing of toxins from the body. This is accomplished in three ways: perspiration, urination, and defecation.

dominatrix   A woman who works with clients, usually male, using bondage, discipline, and other expressions of sadism and masochism for sexual arousal and fantasy fulfillment. She may incorporate certain elements, such as psychodrama, role-playing, and control games.

enzymes   Metabolic protein molecules that catalyze or accelerate every biochemical reaction in the body. There is no life without enzymes.

exfoliation   The casting off or coming off in flakes, scales, or layers—as skin, bark, etc.

feng shui   The ancient Chinese art of placement determines the arrangement of furnishings and accessories to encourage the maximum flow of energy, known as *chi,* and to create ultimate harmony.

free radicals   Unstable molecules with unpaired electrons in their outer shell. They seek to steal an electron from other molecules, setting off a chain reaction of cellular destruction, destroying healthy cells in the process.

gerontology   The scientific study of the aging process and the problems of aging people.

gluten   A gray, sticky substance found in the flour of wheat and other grains that gives dough its tough, elastic quality. Intolerance to gluten has been implicated in a wide variety of allergies.

homeopathy   A complete system of complementary medicine based on the principle that "like cures like." It was developed by a German physician, Samuel Hahnemann (1755–1843), who formulated medicines that create a condition that is similar to the illness; this causes the body to defend itself against the pathology. As the body's defenses are activated, they work to cure the disease.

humectants   These attract moisture to the skin's surface and hold it there. These moisturizing agents slow aging by making the skin softer and preventing dryness and chapping. Natural humectants include honey, which also has antibacterial properties, and aloe vera, which has natural healing properties. Both can be used to treat everything from dry skin, burns, inset bites, and heat rash to acne, cuts, and abrasions.

lipofuscin   The liver-colored brown markings on the skin that are commonly called age spots. They appear all over the body, especially in areas that are exposed to the sun.

mantra A word or phrase that is used as a mental focal point to prevent the mind from distracting thoughts. A mantra can also be used as a specific positive force against negative thinking.

meridians Channels throughout the body through which qi—energy—flows. Energy blockages at the points where these meridians intersect can be released through acupuncture and acupressure massage.

metabolism The rate at which the body transforms food, air, and other nutrients into a form that it can use to function properly through a series of chemical processes. These functions have taken the blame for many an extra pound and a whole lot of excuses for overeating and laziness. Excuses aside, sluggish metabolism can become a real concern as you age; it can be diagnosed easily and remedied by diet and exercise changes, however.

nonfoods We coined this term to distinguish foods that are nutritionally deficient or deleterious to health, reserving the term "food" solely for those elements that enhance the health of the body.

ophthalmologists Medical doctors who specialize in diseases and surgery of the eyes.

optometrists Trained and licensed practitioners who test vision and prescribe corrective lenses. Optometrists earn a doctorate but are not medical doctors.

orthodontia The dental specialty concerned with correcting irregularities in the teeth by bringing the teeth into proper alignment. This is accomplished by using wires and bands to move the teeth into place.

osteopathy The medical practice that incorporates manipulation of the bones to treat ailments which are believed to result from the pressure of displaced bones on nerves.

phytonutrients Intensely rich nutritional elements with outstanding healing properties. Found only in edible plants.

prebiotics Specific carbohydrates that serve as fertilizer to nourish the positive strains of bacteria that are battling disease. *Fructooligo saccharides* (*FOS*) are potent prebiotics that taste like sugar syrup but are not metabolized as sugar and are non-glycemic.

probiotics Colonies of microorganisms present in the intestines that combat unhealthy bacterial growth. These friendly bacteria are considered a second immune system.

qi To the Chinese, *qi*—or *chi*—is the living energy that sustains all life. This energy moves throughout the body along a network of channels or meridians. The points where these channels intersect can be stimulated to free blockages that slow the passage of qi through the channels so that all organs and tissue receive the power needed for the body to function at top potential.

311

qi kung   A 3,000-year-old Chinese healing exercise discipline, *qi kung* combines slow, precise movements; powerful, controlled breathing; and sounds that remove energy blockages and increase the flow of blood and qi to all vital organs.

reflexology   The art of foot massage that manipulates areas of the feet that correspond to organs in the body to promote balance and healing.

RetroAge™   Hattie trademarked and registered the word *RetroAge* to introduce a paradigm shift in the way we view aging. She hopes it will become part of the English language to bring consciousness to the possibility of aging in reverse. It will appear in the dictionary as a verb: *RetroAge* (v.t.) the act of aging in reverse.

sebum   The waxy substance produced by minute glands embedded in the skin, the *sebaceous glands*. Sebum helps to keep the skin's surface supple and prevents it from drying out. When the glands in the scalp are overproductive, hair has an oily appearance. When the buildup of sebum hardens, blood flow through the scalp is slowed, which weakens hair at the root.

starve-and-stuff syndrome   A term we coined to describe the pattern of severely restrictive dieting to lose weight (starving), followed by periods of rapid weight gain caused from massive overeating (stuffing).

super-dense nutrients (SDNs)   Natural whole foods that are rich in essential fatty acids, protein, enzymes, and minerals that provide the body with all the raw materials—phytonutrients—necessary for building youth and maintaining a healthy, fit body for a lifetime.

synovial fluid   The motor oil that keeps our joints moving smoothly and without friction. Produced by the synovium membrane that surrounds our joints or tendons. It not only lubricates surrounding surfaces but also nourishes these tissues.

tantric sex   A style of making love that is Hindu in origin, *tantric sex* concentrates on the eroticism of the entire body. It requires that the male hold back from ejaculation for an extended period of time while the couple continues to pleasure each other without concentrating solely on the genitals.

temporomandibular joints (TMJs)   Located on both sides of the face, these joints connect the movable lower jaw—the mandible—to the stationary bones of the skull. These joints act as hinges, allowing the mouth to open and close. Any dysfunction in the TMJs can cause headaches and severe neck and jaw pain, especially when opening the mouth wide. This is known as *temporomandibular joint syndrome*. People who have this condition often hear clicking and popping sounds and frequently experience a deviation of the jaw upon opening their mouths.

transitionals   On the path of refining one's diet, a person may find there are still some items that are difficult to eliminate all at once. Ultimately, these *transitionals* will be excluded from a healthy diet.

Index

319